GLOBAL HEALTH IN PRACTICE

Investing Amidst Pandemics,
Denial of Evidence,
and Neo-dependency

World Scientific Series in Health Investment and Financing

ISSN: 2591-7315

Series Editor: Alexander S. Preker *(Columbia University, USA and Health Investment & Financing Corp, USA)*

Most western developed countries offer universal access to healthcare through mechanisms that provide financial protection against its high cost, either through insurance or government subsidy programs.

In most middle- and low-income countries, financing is often at the center of reforms in the healthcare sector. Success or failure of these reforms can have major impact on the political survival of governments that get involved, and major implications for the dynamics of the healthcare industry and overall economy.

With this series, World Scientific will contribute knowledge about a policy area which is still poorly-understood. The series merges policy and practice, exploring the economic underpinnings of real trends in health investment and financing.

The series will appeal and be accessible to investors, the health insurance industry, healthcare actuaries, business schools with healthcare tracts, healthcare management programs, researchers, graduate students, policy makers and practitioners working in the health sector worldwide.

More information on this series can also be found at https://www.worldscientific.com/series/wsshif

(Continued at end of book)

World Scientific Series in Health Investment and Financing – Vol. 6

GLOBAL HEALTH IN PRACTICE

Investing Amidst Pandemics, Denial of Evidence, and Neo-dependency

OLUSOJI ADEYI

Resilient Health Systems, USA
Johns Hopkins University, USA

World Scientific

NEW JERSEY · LONDON · SINGAPORE · BEIJING · SHANGHAI · HONG KONG · TAIPEI · CHENNAI · TOKYO

Published by

World Scientific Publishing Co. Pte. Ltd.

5 Toh Tuck Link, Singapore 596224

USA office: 27 Warren Street, Suite 401-402, Hackensack, NJ 07601

UK office: 57 Shelton Street, Covent Garden, London WC2H 9HE

Library of Congress Cataloging-in-Publication Data

Names: Adeyi, Olusoji, author.

Title: Global health in practice : investing amidst pandemics, denial of evidence, and
     neo-dependency / Olusoji Adeyi, Resilient Health Systems, USA, Johns Hopkins University, USA.

Description: New Jersey : World Scientific, 2022. | Series: World scientific series in health
     investment and financing, 2591-7315 ; vol 6 | Includes bibliographical references and index.

Identifiers: LCCN 2021046318 | ISBN 9789811245954 (hardcover) |
     ISBN 9789811245961 (ebook) | ISBN 9789811245978 (ebook other)

Subjects: LCSH: World health. | Public health--International cooperation.

Classification: LCC RA441 .A333 2022 | DDC 362.1962/414--dc23

LC record available at https://lccn.loc.gov/2021046318

British Library Cataloguing-in-Publication Data

A catalogue record for this book is available from the British Library.

ISBN 978-981-125-375-1 (pbk)

For any available supplementary material, please visit
https://www.worldscientific.com/worldscibooks/10.1142/12520#t=suppl

Desk Editors: Aanand Jayaraman/Yulin Jiang

Typeset by Stallion Press
Email: enquiries@stallionpress.com

Printed in Singapore

In memory of
Samuel Adetunji Adeyi
The *Indelible*
(1924–2005)

Foreword

Soji Adeyi and I have known each other and worked together for many years. *Global Health in Practice* reflects three characteristics that, in my experience, characterize Soji: mental agility, candor, and a sense of humor. These characteristics make the book a good read. COVID-19 makes it a timely read — timely not because the book is appearing in the course of the pandemic, but rather because COVID-19 has exposed deep shortcomings in institutions and practices. And it is precisely these problems (and the long history underlying them) that *Global Health in Practice* addresses. Soji's own career as a practitioner — from serving as a young doctor in Nigeria to working at senior levels of the World Bank — provides him with a breadth of perspective that few can match. This practical experience combined with his wide reading has led to a book rich in context and provocative in message.

The book's intention is not only to provoke thought but also to point to achievable reform. The book argues that "...complexity is not an excuse for paralysis amidst vast unmet needs...." Taking this to heart Soji makes his core conclusions clear. What are these conclusions? Two of the most important are:

First, *end foreign aid for basic health inputs.* Vaccination, treatment of common diseases, and the supply chain capacity behind them are "...so highly cost-effective and the need for them is so predictable that they should be elementary responsibilities for the countries themselves." This transition in foreign-aid practice would be radical and Soji thus argues for an 8-year period to allow countries the time to assume these responsibilities for themselves.

Second, the transition Soji argues for is not a transition away from foreign aid but rather a transition to where added value is high. There are many dimensions to this transition but the core direction is toward financing *global and regional public* goods like creation and transfer of knowledge, and for preparation at country, regional, and global levels for unpredictable events like COVID-19.

Soji's conclusions are indeed clear, and implementation would go a long way toward addressing the problems that the book exposes and dissects. But the conclusions are as radical as they are clear. Conservative opposition is inevitable.

The book opens with reflections on the angst in global health, followed by an incisive exploration of the strategic and geopolitical lessons from the COVID-19 pandemic. It then provides a primer on the roles of governments and markets in health, setting the stage for two illustrative chapters. One is about a large public–private partnership to improve access to malaria medicines, which Soji examines from his vantage point as director of the enterprise that translated the concept into practice. Careful independent evaluation of the malaria experience appears in *The Lancet*, with strongly positive conclusions, but the result exemplified Soji's concern about aversion to evidence. USAID representatives killed the partnership despite both the evidence and the clear preference of officials from malaria endemic countries to continue.

Soji comes to this book with unusually deep experiences in different parts of the world, as shown in his astute examinations of health policy and practice during the political and economic transitions of health in Russia and Nigeria. Through these examples, he guides the reader through the convergence of the technocratic and political dimensions of health leadership in practice.

The chapter on the realities of development assistance for health is a masterclass on the complex realities of that wide-ranging aspect of global health. Soji discusses the issues with his characteristic candor. The illustrative vignettes bring to life the real-life dynamics of an important dimension of global health: the interplay of incentives created and experienced by financiers from the Global North, governments of the Global South, and their agents.

Beyond presenting new ways of looking at long-standing and vexing problems, this book challenges the reader to think and act differently when seeking solutions to those problems. While recognizing the legacy of colonialism and current injustices in the architecture of global health, Soji posits that the real problem is not neo-colonialism, but neo-dependency. In this, he seeks to change the direction and focus of much energy and discourse in global health. It is a central challenge for current and future policy makers, scholars, practitioners, and investors in global health.

Financiers of health innovations and programs, whether from domestic or external sources, can learn much from this book. Policy makers and their advisors will find clear directions for reform. Academics will find it handy in bridging the gap between theory and practice. Students will have a companion as they prepare to study and then influence both policy and practice in global health. For its strategic relevance, candor, and depth of insight, this timely book is a must-read.

Dean T. Jamison
Edward A. Clarkson Professor, Emeritus
University of California, San Francisco

Preface

In the introduction to *A History of Global Health*, Professor Randall Packard reflects on the complexities of choosing between options for improving health, noting that arguments could be made for moving in different directions. He notes that decisions are often shaped by intricate historical circumstances and stresses the importance of understanding these forces and how they have defined and limited global health interventions. His book has a subtitle: *Interventions into the Lives of Other Peoples*. I imagine that were that book cowritten by Walter Rodney,[a] he might have called it *How the Global North Under-Developed Health Systems in the Global South*. The composite Packard-Rodney subtitle, though imaginary, is reflected in parts of this book, but it is far from being the meta-narrative. Had I coauthored that same book, while addressing history without flinching, we might have discussed the bigger picture, with a subtitle that is both averse to a narrative of victimhood and heavy on responsibility: *How the Global South Condemns Itself to Neo-Dependency*.

This book is an explorer's guide to global health in real life, with attention to the dynamics in three interrelated theaters: within the Global North, at the North-South interface, and within the Global South. The past century mostly was a period of marked improvements in health outcomes. Humanity now faces multiple challenges: delivering on the heady

---

[a]Walter Anthony Rodney (1942–1980) was the author of *How Europe Underdeveloped Africa*.

promises of Universal Health Coverage (UHC) amidst resource constraints; ensuring Global Health Security amidst a fractured architecture of global health and diplomacy; and optimizing global trade for collective interests in a world where the primordial self-interests of the Global North run contrary to such solidarity.

In the foregoing context, the COVID-19 pandemic has laid bare the greatest geopolitical lesson of the early 21st century for countries of the Global South: in moments of great peril, they cannot count on the rich countries of the Global North for timely and equity-based collective action. The Global North would be forthcoming only as a last resort, and only after much obfuscation and foot dragging. Since health is a matter of national security and a bedrock of global security, the production and distribution of strategic medical equipment, drugs, and vaccines are too important to be left to the market alone; governments should strategically and selectively invest in industrial production and supply chains. While it is a global catastrophe, the COVID-19 pandemic itself is not the fundamental problem. It merely reveals long-running flaws of conception, design, execution, and failures to learn in global health.

Current and potential investors can hardly avoid vexing questions about the roles of markets, the private sector, and governments in global health. Discussions about markets and governments often evoke strongly held beliefs and positions, particularly on appropriate roles of the private sector and public policy. While reasonable people might hold different viewpoints, the facts indicate that ideological purity, whether for or against the market, is an imprudent stance. It is important to look at — and beyond — the failures of governments and markets, with attention to just what it is that decision makers are optimizing for. Doing so paves the way for measured considerations of equity of access to technologies and services, and for careful distinctions between means and ends.

Real-life cases provide insight into the policy dynamics, political vagaries, and gritty aspects of global health at country level. The Affordable Medicines Facility for Malaria (AMFm) illustrates the good, the bad, and the despicable of global health architecture in practice. It offers a glimpse of what is possible with the power of new ideas, the willingness to try new ways of solving long-standing problems, and a coalition that is willing to subject a new approach to the glare of a rigorous independent evaluation. It also illustrates the perils of having *de facto* veto powers in the hands of any single hegemonic financier whose fealty to a *status quo* stifled innovation and scuppered evidence-based changes that would benefit millions of people. In this case, the United States Agency for International Development (USAID) and the United States President's Malaria Initiative (US-PMI) were the fundamental obstacles to progress.

The Southern Africa region illustrates the combined effects of unbridled capitalist exploitation and political inheritance on modern-day health policies. This case study goes beyond the "what" and the "how" to examine the "why" of policy dynamics in the region, and in the country of South Africa in particular. Such understanding, which explains — but neither justifies nor excuses — apparent irrationalities and injustices in health systems, is a precondition for effective leadership in seemingly impossible situations. It opens a window into the case for restorative justice after decades of state-sanctioned policies that explicitly discounted the humanity and health of the majority.

Political and economic transitions can put additional stress on already resource-constrained health systems. Russia experienced severe stress during its tumultuous transition from the Soviet era. The account in this book unpacks the dynamics of science, politics, and controversies around investing in tuberculosis (TB) and HIV/AIDS control in the immediate post-Soviet Russian Federation. The challenge was to successfully negotiate with Russia an agreement to combine technical guidelines from the World Health Organization (WHO) with financing from an external multilateral development financier — the World Bank — for a large program to curb the dual epidemics of TB and HIV/AIDS. It is a first-hand account of an interplay of political history, science, incongruent geopolitical cues, and ultimate resolution in the direction of progress.

Nigeria's health system is caught in the dynamics of economic transition from LIC to LMIC status. That transition lays bare the interactions among political history, contemporary policies, financing, health status, the domestic political economy, and the engagement between country-based experts and their external counterparts. Central to this case study is that wallowing in the past is not the solution to current problems, as that would not only absolve recent and current policy makers of responsibility but also infantilize and deny the agency of the population. The case links several factors at play: the realities of Nigeria's quest for UHC through a viable health system; the dynamics of legislation, budgeting, and implementation; the realities of Development Assistance for Health (DAH); and opportunities for better performance. It combines empirical data with attention to the functions of institutions and to the compact — or lack of same — between the government and the governed in matters of health.

Have financiers from the Global North used DAH to recolonize the Global South? DAH presumes common interests, with particular benefit for the recipients, to be enabled by a net flow of knowledge, know-how, and financial resources from the Global North to the Global South. Implicit in that construct are assumptions of a net superiority of the Global North in the production of better health for the Global South. Those assumptions have damaging implications in practice. The dynamics play out through multiple transactions and bargaining among centers of influence, power, and perceived powerlessness in global health. While DAH has many positives, it also has enormous dysfunction. The din of protest against colonialism in global health is getting louder and it has merit. However, I posit that the deeper problem is the neo-dependency of the Global South on the Global North. The responsibility for self-release from that bondage falls on the Global South.

A frank treatise on ending neo-dependency is the unspoken third rail of global health. It is a taboo, usually mentioned *sotto voce* and only in the most circuitous euphemisms, lest powerful sensitivities be offended. A frontal assault on neo-dependency is hazardous for two reasons. First, by removing the veneer of charity that disguises the debilitating aspects of foreign aid, it raises the ire of the Foreign Aid Industrial Complex — especially but not only bilateral financiers beholden to the *status quo*, and a parasitic subset of NGOs from the Global North. Second, by challenging the Global South to take charge of its own destiny, it raises questions about which institutional and individual entities in the Global South perpetuate and benefit from self-subjugation and the lack of accountability of governments to their populations. Nevertheless, neo-dependency must be addressed in stark terms, and it must end, if the Global South is to emancipate itself from long-running subservience in global health.

There is a need for bold changes in the architecture and dynamics of global health. The trend toward neo-dependency needs to stop, as does the gaming of development assistance by the Global North and the Global South. How can local investors — governments and the private sector alike — maximize the health and institutional impacts of their investments in LICs and MICs? How can external investors — donors and private sector alike — be assured of more value for money, transparency, and brighter prospects for not being needed for indefinite periods? What will it take to change the metasystem through which the Global North condescendingly — and often disingenuously — dictates what the Global South must do? Fundamental changes would upend global health practice as we know it and they are sure to draw the ire of guardians of the *status quo*.

Enduring pearls of wisdom from Professor Chinua Achebe's *Anthills of the Savannah* come to mind:

> *"Charity, he thundered, is the opium of the privileged; from the good citizen who habitually drops ten kobo from his loose change and from a safe height above the bowl of the leper outside the supermarket; to the group of good citizens like yourselves who donate water so that some Lazarus in the slums can have a syringe boiled clean as a whistle for his jab and his sores dressed more hygienically than the rest of him; to the Band Aid stars that lit up so dramatically the dark Christmas skies of Ethiopia. While we do our good works let us not forget that the real solution lies in a world in which charity will have become unnecessary."*

To those who would seek to justify or perpetuate the *status quo*, and to those who would rather continue endless rounds of cosmetic reforms, meetings that lead nowhere, and hollow rituals of ineffectual declarations, the question is: *cui bono?*

Olusoji Adeyi

About the Author

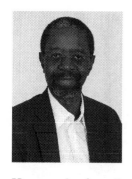 **Dr. Olusoji (Soji) Adeyi** is the President of Resilient Health Systems, a policy analysis and advisory services firm based in Washington DC, and a Senior Associate at the Johns Hopkins Bloomberg School of Public Health in Baltimore. In his prior career at the World Bank, he served as Director of the Health, Nutrition, and Population Global Practice and as Senior Advisor for Human Development, among other leadership responsibilities across the world. He was the founding Director of the Affordable Medicines Facility for malaria at the Global Fund to Fight AIDS, Tuberculosis, and Malaria. Dr. Adeyi served as Associate Director of the AIDS Prevention Initiative in Nigeria, which was funded by the Bill and Melinda Gates Foundation through the Harvard School of Public Health. He has led many initiatives on global health policies, strategies, and programs across the world. He has also had responsibilities with the Federal Ministry of Health in Nigeria, WHO, and UNAIDS. He has authored many papers and books on health policy, health systems, service delivery, quality of care, maternal health, health financing, disease control, and pollution.

Dr. Adeyi has co-led and shaped multiple partnerships and studies in global health, including as a Board member of the Stop TB Partnership, the Roll Back Malaria Partnership, the TB Alliance (a not-for-profit product development partnership), and Last Mile Health; as a member of The Advisory Committee to the Editors of Disease Control Priorities,

3rd Edition; and as a member of The International Task Force for Disease Eradication. He served as a Commissioner on The Lancet Global Health Commission on High Quality Health Systems and The Lancet Commission on Pollution and Health.

Dr. Adeyi was born in Nigeria, where he earned his bachelor's degree with first class honors and his medical degree with honors at the University of Ife. His postgraduate education includes Master of Community Health from the Liverpool School of Tropical Medicine — where he was a Rotary Foundation Scholar, Master of Business Administration from Imperial College London and the University of London, and Doctor of Public Health from the Johns Hopkins University in Baltimore.

Webpage: www.ResilientHealthSystems.com

Twitter: @sojiadeyi

Acknowledgments

In my mind, I have written variants of this book over and over, but never found the time to put them on paper. Alexander S. Preker, editor-in-chief of the World Scientific Series in Health Investment and Financing, catalyzed my decision to write it at this time, and he provided valuable insight and practical help along the way.

I have had extraordinary opportunities to work with and learn from innumerable leaders, policy makers, researchers, program managers, partners, hecklers, journalists, colleagues, and friends all over the world. For the combination of experiences and knowledge that informed my approach to this book, I am indebted to them all as my teachers in the broadest sense of the word. They bear no responsibility for this book. In fact, a plenary discussion of the book would feature spirited debates — and many collegial disagreements!

"Green P. Decroly," the anonymous reviewer of the entire manuscript, is a gem of inestimable value. For critical and helpful comments on all or some draft chapters, I thank Anne Bakilana, Enis Baris, Mickey Chopra, Maria Gracheva, Dean Jamison, Shunsuke Mabuchi, Ronald Mutasa, Yuniwo Nfor, Oluwole Odutolu, Olumide Okunola, and Gaston Sorgho. The reviewers were immensely helpful. While thanking them, I absolve them of any responsibility for the contents of the book or any error therein.

Fela, the wheaten terrier, was my inseparable companion during the writing of this book and he heard much about global health during many video calls. The time spent writing featured mood music by Wynton

Marsalis, Cannonball Adderley, Jimmy Smith, John Coltrane, Miles Davis, Charlie Parker, B.B. King, Ella Fitzgerald, Cesária Évora, Luis Fonsi, Grover Washington, Jr., Stanley Turrentine, Duke Ellington, Bob James, The Dave Brubeck Quartet, Hank Crawford, Bob Marley, Ebenezer Obey, King Sunny Ade, Victor Uwaifo, Sade Adu, Enya, Stevie Wonder, Davido, Kassav, Fela Anikulapo-Kuti, Miriam Makeba, Hugh Masekela, The Beatles, Ray Charles, Louis Armstrong, Quincy Jones, Kenny Rogers, and Zaiko Langa Langa.

Enormous thanks are due to the editorial, production, and promotion teams at World Scientific Publishing. I appreciate the work of Nisha Das, Aanand Jayaraman, Jiang Yulin, Lee Hooi Yean, and all their colleagues who made this publication possible.

Writing a book is very fulfilling and instructive. It can also be a lonely journey. I am especially grateful for the moral support and encouragement from my wife Gabriella, and sons Nicholas and Michael.

Thank you.

Contents

List of Figures

List of Tables

List of Boxes

List of Composite Vignettes

List of Acronyms

ACT	Artemisinin-Based Combination Therapy
ACT Accelerator	Access to COVID-19 Tools Accelerator
AIDS	Acquired Immune Deficiency Syndrome
ALMA	African Leaders Malaria Alliance
AMFm	Affordable Medicines Facility for malaria
AMRH	African Medicines Regulatory Harmonization Initiative
AMT	Artemisinin Monotherapy
AU	African Union
AUDA	African Union Development Agency
AVAREF	African Vaccine Regulatory Forum
AVATT	African Vaccine Acquisition Task Team
BCC	Behavior Change Communication
BMGF	Bill and Melinda Gates Foundation
BMPHS	Basic Minimum Package of Health Services
CCM	Country Coordinating Mechanism
CDC	Centers for Disease Control and Prevention
CHAI	Clinton Health Access Initiative
CIDA	Canadian International Development Agency
CIS	Commonwealth of Independent States

COIDA	Compensation for Occupational Injuries and Diseases Act
COVAX	COVID-19 Vaccines Global Access
COVID-19	The disease caused by a new coronavirus called SARS-CoV-2
CQ	Chloroquine
CRDH	Centre de Recherche pour le Developpement Humain
CSW	Commercial Sex Worker
CT	Computerized tomography
CTAG	Copayment Technical Advisory Group
DAH	Development Assistance for Health
DANIDA	Danish International Development Agency
DDT	Dichloro-diphenyl-trichloroethane
DEC	Development Economics Research Group of the World Bank
DFID	Department for International Development (United Kingdom)
DHS	Demographic and Health Survey
DLI	Disbursement-Linked Indicator
DNDi	Drugs for Neglected Diseases initiative
DOTS	Directly Observed Treatment — Short Course
DPs	Development Partners
EMT	Economic Management Team
EMT	Emergency Medical Treatment
EU	European Union
FIND	Foundation for Innovative New Diagnostics
FMOH	Federal Ministry of Health
FRWG	Finance and Resources Working Group (of RBM)
Gavi	Gavi, The Vaccine Alliance
GDP	Gross Domestic Product

GFATM	Global Fund to Fight AIDS, Tuberculosis, and Malaria
GIS	Geographic Information System
GMP	Global Malaria Program (of the World Health Organization)
GMP	Good Manufacturing Practices
GNI	Gross National Income
GPEI	Global Polio Eradication Initiative
GPS	Global Positioning System
GRZ	Government of the Republic of Zambia
HIC	High-Income Country
HIV	Human Immunodeficiency Virus
HPNSDP	Health, Population, and Nutrition Sector Development Program
HRIP	Health Reform Implementation Project
HLWG	High-Level Working Group
IBRD	International Bank for Reconstruction and Development
IDA	International Development Association
IDU	Injecting Drug User
IEC	Information, Education, and Communication
IFC	International Finance Corporation
IHR	International Health Regulations
IMF	International Monetary Fund
IOM	Institute of Medicine of the National Academies (United States)
IP	Intellectual Property
JICA	Japanese International Cooperation Agency
LGHA	Local Government Health Authority
LIC	Low-Income Country
LMIC	Lower Middle Income Country
LSHTM	London School of Hygiene and Tropical Medicine

MAP	Multicountry AIDS Program in the Africa Region
MBOD	Medical Bureau for Occupational Diseases
MDC	Market Dynamics Committee
MDR-TB	Multidrug-Resistant Tuberculosis
MIC	Middle-Income Country
MICS	Multiple Indicator Cluster Surveys
MMR	Maternal Mortality Ratio
MRI	Magnetic Resonance Imaging
NBHSS	National Basic Health Services Scheme
NEPAD	New Partnership for African Development
NGN	Nigerian Naira
NGO	Non-Governmental Organization
NHIS	National Health Insurance Scheme
NMFI	Non-Malaria Febrile Illness
NPHCDA	National Primary Health Care Development Agency
NPV	Net Present Value
NSIA	Nigeria Sovereign Investment Authority
NSHIP	Nigeria State Health Investment Project
ODA	Official Development Assistance
OECD	Organisation for Economic Co-operation and Development
OLD	Occupational Lung Diseases
OOP	Out-of-Pocket Expenditures
PCR	Polymerase Chain Reaction
PEPFAR	United States President's Emergency Plan For AIDS Relief
PHC	Primary Health Care
PHEIC	Public Health Emergency of International Concern
PPP	Public–Private Partnership
PSC	Policy and Strategy Committee of the Global Fund to Fight AIDS, Tuberculosis, and Malaria Board

PSC	Professional Services Council
PSI	Population Services International
QAACT	Quality-Assured Artemisinin-Based Combination Therapy
RBM	Roll Back Malaria Partnership
RDT	Rapid Diagnostic Test
SADC	Southern African Development Community
SARS-CoV-2	Severe acute respiratory syndrome coronavirus 2
SDGs	Sustainable Development Goals
SIDA	Swedish International Development Cooperation Agency
SP	Sulfadoxine-Pyrimethamine
SPHCB/As	State Primary Health Care Boards/Authorities
SSES	State Sanitary Epidemiological Surveillance
SSHIA	State Social Health Insurance Agency/Scheme
SWAp	Sector-Wide Approach
TB	Tuberculosis
TEBA	Employment Bureau of Africa
TFR	Total Fertility Rate
TIMS	Southern Africa Tuberculosis in the Mining Sector Initiative
TRIPS	Trade-Related Aspects of Intellectual Property
U5MR	Under-five mortality rate
UHC	Universal Health Coverage
UMIC	Upper Middle Income Country
UNAIDS	Joint United Nations Program on HIV/AIDS
UNGA	United Nations General Assembly
UNICEF	United Nations Children's Fund
UNITAID	Global health initiative established by the governments of Brazil, Chile, France, Norway, and the United Kingdom
USAID	United States Agency for International Development

US-CDC   United States Centers for Disease Control and
                Prevention
US-PMI   United States President's Malaria Initiative
WDC   Ward Development Committee
WHO   World Health Organization
WTO   World Trade Organization

Chapter 1

Global Health and Its Congenital Discontents

*"And so, dear boy, I made it home from Troy, in total ignorance,
knowing nothing of their fates, the ones who stayed behind:
who escaped with their lives and who went down.
But all I've gathered by hearsay, sitting here in my own house –
That you'll learn, it's only right, I'll hide nothing now."*

—Homer: *The Odyssey*[a]

Synopsis

This book is about the practice of global health in real life. Global health policy is at a crossroads, especially in the more resource-constrained low-income countries (LICs) and middle-income countries (MICs). It is on trial at the interface between the Global North and the Global South. There has been remarkable progress in multiple dimensions of health outcomes over the past century.[1] Yet, countries face a complex landscape of lofty ambitions in the form of political commitments to universal health coverage (UHC), human capital, and global health security. These ambitions are tempered, implicitly if not explicitly, by severe resource constraints in LICs and MICs, weaknesses in the use of scientific evidence

---

[a]Homer. 1996. *The Odyssey*. Translated by Robert Fagles. New York: Viking Penguin. p. 113.

as the basis for rational policy decisions, gaps in the available science, modest-to-bleak prospects for increases in official development assistance (ODA) in general and development assistance for health (DAH) in particular, suboptimal dynamics of DAH, and ineffectual global health leadership — particularly for global health security. Current and potential investors in global health must navigate a minefield of remarkable but very uneven progress, great expectations, and denials of scientific evidence by entrenched interests. That terrain is further complicated by the hegemonic suppression of innovation that threatens the *status quo* and by self-perpetuating cycles of dependency of the Global South on the Global North.

1.1. The Premise of Global Health in Development

Investing in global health is based on expectations of positive health and system-strengthening returns on investment, common interests in curbing negative externalities of disease outbreaks, and shared sociopolitical interests at the global level. Historical aversions to ill health have morphed into a more positive perception of health as the foundation of wealth, such as the maxim attributed to Ralph Waldo Emerson: "The first wealth is health."[2] The establishment in 1948 of the World Health Organization marked a formal declaration of intent in the post-World War II era, with its idealism of attaining the highest possible state of health for all.[3] Why, amidst the idealism and pressing needs in global health, is it essential to recall and understand its history? Doing so fosters strategic situation awareness because the imperialist origins of global health were neither abstract nor finite in their consequences. Rather, they were rooted in the geopolitical and commercial self-interests of their time, and those themes remain relevant today. Those interests were often lethal for the "natives" of the then colonies and the consequences persist both structurally and functionally. A brief exploration will suffice for this opening chapter.

Rudyard Kipling's *The White Man's Burden*[4] encapsulates the colonial origins and imperialist ancestry of what is now called global health. It exhorted the invader to carry the yoke for civilizing the "half devil and half child" natives in a mission that included curing the sick. Randall Packard[5] examined in detail the colonial origins of global health, social medicine, and rural hygiene, the changing post-World War II visions of health and development, the era of eradication, the population dimensions of global health concerns, the rise and fall of primary health care, and prospects for the future. His work is a must-read for practitioners who seek to understand and influence policies and programs in global health, with particular attention to the dimensions of its subtitle of "Interventions into the lives of other peoples."

How did imperialism and colonialism become founding pillars of global health? There are pointers from the transatlantic slave trade and its close association with the origins of schools of tropical medicine. Many port cities and individuals profited from the business of shipping people into slavery. One such city was Liverpool in England, the origin of ships that carried about 20% of African captives across the Atlantic. As the city saw increasing numbers of people admitted into hospitals because of "tropical diseases," Alfred Jones, a shipping merchant, donated £350 to found the venerable Liverpool School of Tropical Medicine in 1898. The school would investigate the disease outbreaks.[6] Ronald Ross was the school's pioneering teacher in Tropical Medicine and he won a Nobel Prize for his work on the transmission of malaria. In 1901, Alfred Jones, who invested in the mass shipment of humans into bondage, was knighted by King Edward VII "in recognition of services to the West African Colonies, and to Jamaica."[7] He became Sir Alfred Jones. The London Gazette, which recorded the honor, did not include peer-reviewed customer satisfaction surveys of the people whom Sir Jones's ships transported in chains across the Atlantic.

The original London School of Tropical Medicine, which started operations six months after the Liverpool School, was structured with deference to the interests, concerns, and politics of the British Empire as formulated by Joseph Chamberlain, the Colonial Secretary.[8] The British Treasury gave the school financial support, "which was promptly recouped from the indigent colonies."[9]

Not to be outdone, Belgium's King Leopold II in 1906 established a school devoted to the study of tropical diseases in Brussels, which later merged with another institution and moved to Antwerp to form the Institute of Tropical Medicine.[10] King Leopold II wanted to train doctors and nurses to work in the Congo Free State, a vast territory the size of

Western Europe, to which he laid claim. King Leopold II, in whose name heinous crimes against humanity were committed in the Congo, was much admired throughout Europe as a "philanthropic" monarch.[11] Sir Alfred Jones and King Leopold II were not mere celebrities. They were the early 20th century's exemplars of philanthrocapitalism in tropical medicine and they lacked nothing apart from the internet. In contemporary affairs, the inherent contradictions and vexations of such philanthrocapitalism are to be found in works such as *Philanthrocapitalism*[12] and *Winners Take All*.[13]

These roots of global health as we now know it were not confined to the Atlantic theater. The Netherlands has a deep history in colonization, including the Dutch East Indies, now Indonesia. It was also active in the business of enslaving other people. A combination of government and private businesses working in the Dutch colonies founded the KIT Royal Tropical Institute in Amsterdam in 1910. In studying the tropics and fostering trade in the colonies, its mission was cast as serving supposedly shared interests of the colonizer and the colonized:

> *"... a particular worldview, one best summarized by the words of Queen Wilhemina (sic) on the day of the building's opening in 1926: 'Above all, this proud building voices the depth and certainty of our conviction that the interests and needs of the East and West Indies are the same as those of the Netherlands.' Since then, the certainty of this conviction has faded as new worldviews emerged in the post-colonial era."*[14]

Straining to define shared needs and interests of the colonized and to romanticize the conditions of the enslaved were common during the era of colonization and slavery. James Penny, a slave trader in Liverpool, once asserted that "The slaves here will sleep better than the gentlemen do on shore."[15] Nobody at the time conducted a randomized controlled trial of the effects of slavery on sleeping conditions.

The United States of America, through its colonial possessions in the Caribbean, Panama, and the Philippines, contributed to the construct that formed both the structures and narratives of international health in the 20th century. There are enduring impacts of investments made by the Rockefeller Foundation in the early 20th century. In 1913, the foundation created an International Health Commission, which was renamed the

International Health Board (IHB) in 1916 and renamed the International Health Division (IHD) in 1927. By the time it folded in 1951, it had operated in 80 countries, fighting tropical diseases and financing the establishment of schools of tropical medicine and public health. In the United States, the schools included those at the Johns Hopkins University and Harvard University. The Rockefeller Foundation also funded other schools of public health in 21 countries and trained hundreds of health professionals from developing countries.[5] The goals of sanitizing the world and advancing western civilization were intertwined.

1.2. The Expedient Advent of Development Assistance for Global Health

What is now called global health evolved from the health brigade of the colonizer's task force to conquer and civilize *the natives*. That health brigade mitigated some of the risks of investors' bets on imperial expeditions. The transformation from colonial functions to combinations of foreign aid and technical assistance took off after World War II and the disintegration of empires. For example, in the Netherlands, the government sought new ways to keep its former colonial servants engaged and to claw back its global influence. "In the 1960s, Dutch development aid expanded enormously and changed in nature. It became much less focused on (former) Dutch colonies and changed from being idealistically motivated to being more motivated by pragmatic Dutch self-interest."[16] Despite the country's history of industrial-scale involvement in slavery, the Netherlands has yet to foster an open reckoning with the meaning and consequences of that aspect of its past.[17]

There emerged a network of institutions and individuals who combined teaching and research with support for preventing and treating diseases that threatened the returns on investments made by colonial and postcolonial powers across the world. Those institutions have made — and continue to make — outstanding contributions to knowledge. They have trained generations of experts across the world in tropical medicine and public health. Their faculty have worked in some of the most challenging locations the world over. Professionals trained in those schools have made stellar contributions to research, teaching, and practice. Those are extraordinary achievements that have made the world a better place by pushing the frontiers of knowledge in public health and medicine.

In tandem with the stellar intellectual contributions of those institutions and individuals, colonialism planted the seed of a construct that persists today: the Global North decides the narrative and assumes the omniscience to tell the Global South what the latter needs, when it can have it, how to do it, and on whose terms it must be done. More importantly, it laid the foundation for a system that combined a claim of omnipotence (through the *power* of colonizers) with a claim of omniscience (through the *truth* — as emanating from a supposedly benign and knowledge-based network). A monopoly of the combination of power and the truth stifles contestation of the grand narrative. The monopoly is inherently precarious because the colonized never asked to be subjugated. It is also self-destructive because truth, to maintain legitimacy, must strive against power, lest it be reduced to falsehoods that fuel power. Thus, to earn credibility and durable legitimacy in a post-colonial era, the knowledge-based network created by colonialism must repudiate the very ethos of colonialism from which it originated. Such renunciation is a lofty ideal in theory, a romantic quest on social media, and an improbable scenario in real life. The conundrum is not limited to global health. Professor Wole Soyinka[b] paints a broader picture of the problem:

> *"Well, the first thing is that truth and power for me form an antithesis, an antagonism, which will hardly ever be resolved. I can define in fact, can simplify the history of human society, the evolution of human society, as a contest between power and freedom. And whether this contest is being performed along ideological lines or along religious lines, ultimately, really what we have is truth versus power. Truth for me is freedom, is self-destination. Power is domination, control, and therefore a very selective form of truth which is a lie. And the polarity between these two, in fact, forms for me the axis of human striving in the creation of an ethical society, an ethical community."*[18]

---

[b]Wole Soyinka won the Nobel Prize for Literature in 1986.

The power dynamics are evident in today's global health. Contemporary strains of the narrative of what is good for *the natives* persist in some policy circles and through deleterious variants of technical assistance. They run through the assertions by some leaders and institutions of the Global North on what the Global South needs to fight COVID-19 (see Chapter 2), regardless of — and often directly contrary to — what leaders and institutions of the Global South say they need. They underpin the business models of some cash-rich bilateral financiers of health programs, especially the United States Agency for International Development (USAID) and the United States President's Malaria Initiative (US-PMI) (see Chapter 4). They determine much of the dysfunction in DAH (see Chapter 8).

Global health thus came into being with major congenital defects that remain uncorrected. The defects persist partly because their definitive diagnoses are unsettling. They endure because their definitive treatments require major changes in the dominant narratives, structures, and functions that legitimize the *status quo*.

The post-World War II jostling for spheres of influence among the wealthy nations spilled over into foreign aid, channeled through bilateral and multilateral development assistance. Despite the establishment of the WHO, improving health initially was not a universally shared priority for development assistance. For example, the World Bank in its earlier days did not formally regard investing in health as an essential driver of development.[19] Its approach has evolved positively over the past three decades, both qualitatively and quantitatively, into support for UHC.[20] It has made wide-ranging and positive contributions to health through its analyses, policy consultations, and program financing. The evolution and positive contributions have been punctuated by, among others, an initial squeamishness about tackling HIV/AIDS and a recent fiasco of the Pandemic Emergency Facility (PEF).[21] Despite the sound health, economic, and moral rationale for UHC, and despite calls to prioritize UHC amidst the COVID-19 pandemic,[22] it remains to be seen whether UHC is a manifest destiny or a Sisyphean adventure.[23]

The genre of global health gained more insight and traction with Professor John Bryant's *Health and The Developing World*.[24] A *tour de force*, it highlighted tensions among aspirations, standards, resource constraints, and operational realities in the "developing World." In that book, Bryant, with whom I had the privilege of working at the Aga Khan University in Karachi in 1989, wrote the following regarding DAH:

> *"Since there are similarities among developing countries, there is a tendency to lump them together in seeking common solutions to their problems. Actually, many of the problems are similar, such as the diseases, the lack of resources, and the maldistribution of health personnel. The great differences are to be found in the settings of those problems, the culture, the tradition, the economic capability, and the style of handling those problems."*
>
> *"The point is that if donor agencies in the health field want to use their resources in ways most likely to influence the health of a nation, it will take discerning and knowledgeable persons to choose the strategic points of need, and it may require the donor agency to formulate new criteria, even new mechanisms of giving."*
>
> *"To give effectively is an exacting task. To give without doing harm is, surprisingly, equally exacting. This is particularly so when donations are required to be matched in some way by the recipient country."*

Five decades later, and despite more attention to what is now called global health diplomacy,[25,26] Bryant's key messages remain both true and poorly learned by institutions and governments. I posit that the failures to learn arise not from a collective inability to do so, but from unwillingness and outright refusals to do so, as such learning would logically lead to changes that upend the *status quo* of rent seeking in both the Global North and the Global South. The latter bears an additional responsibility because many countries in the Global South have become all too willing to rationalize their dependency on the kindness of strangers from the Global North to finance their basic health services.

There is a discernible but nonlinear progression from colonial health to international health, and to global health. Much has been written about overlaps and distinctions between colonial health, public health, international health, and global health. Koplan *et al.* provide helpful analysis to inform their definition of global health as "an area for study, research, and practice that places a priority on improving health and achieving equity in health for all people worldwide."[27] I use the term *Global Health* in this book to mean *the sum of learning, influencing, practicing, and applying knowledge, know-how, and financing to improve health outcomes and systems globally, with emphasis on equity and social justice.* In this book, the "global" in *Global Health* refers to the spirit of shared habitation on the same planet, of a shared destiny as co-occupants of a single room — albeit a large one, of shared humanity, and an ethos that says *we are all in this together.* It must be noted, however, that the nomenclature remains a matter of some discussion in contemporary academia. For example, the Johns Hopkins University has both a Department of International Health within its Bloomberg School of Public Health[28] and a Center for Global Health.[29]

1.3. Disinvesting and Investing in Global Health

"Ignorance allows people to disregard the consequences of their actions. And sometimes it leads to consequences even they did not intend."

—Michael Lewis[c]

The current momentum for investing in global health derived largely from a convergence of influential research and, paradoxically, a backlash against on-the-ground realities of cuts in publicly financed health services driven by the Structural Adjustment Programs of the 1980s. The International Monetary Fund (IMF) and the World Bank drove those programs. The backlash against Structural Adjustment Program cuts in public funding of health services was loud and enduring. Calls for "Adjustment with a human face" gained traction in the 1980s and 1990s, most loudly through activism and prominent publications from parts of the Global North and through street protests and strikes by those directly affected in the Global South.[30–32]

There are thoughtful reflections on the responses of health systems to structural adjustment.[33] However, there has been no definitive and formal reckoning on the net effects of Structural Adjustment Programs on health

---

[c]Lewis M. 2018. *The Fifth Risk.* New York: W.W. Norton & Company. p. 115.

spending and outcomes,[34] and no definitive and formal reckoning on the influential research that promoted user fees for health services in developing countries.[35,36] Regression equations and models predicated on assumptions of *ceteris paribus* have important uses, but their translation into externally driven policies can be robotically detached from human realities. For analysts who have experienced neither the gritty realities of health workers forced to prematurely discharge from hospitals the patients who could not pay steep user fees, nor seen up close the wrenching choices faced by the families of those patients, it might be hard to appreciate the damage that Structural Adjustment Programs did in real life. A Truth and Reconciliation Summit might be in order.

Investing in Health, the World Bank's influential 1993 World Development Report, triggered waves of public discussions on the rationale for investing in health and technocratic debates about how best to achieve health value for money.[37] It highlighted how much health could be bought for rather modest sums of money. It also highlighted the reality of rationing care; matters that had been subsumed in euphemisms were made explicit. Finally, it raised questions deriving from perceptions of institutional inconsistency on the broader determinants of health, including access to sanitation and potable water.[38] Bloom *et al.*, who estimated a production function of aggregate economic growth including work experience and health as fundamental components of human capital, found that good health had a statistically significant and positive effect on aggregate output.[39]

Investing in Health was a strategist's dream come true in that it had a multiplier effect on discourse, lexicon, and the shaping of resource allocation. It was also a technocrat's delight in its assumption of rationality and linearity in decision-making amidst limited resources. For ideologues who utterly rejected the reality of finite resources amidst competing priorities, and who believed that everyone must be guaranteed every health service, it was the perfect piñata; always full, always intact, and available for bashing over and over. For anyone seeking to inform program options and decisions at the country level, it was a road that led to the sobering reality that health policy makers and politicians would rather ration implicitly than explicitly. The idea of essential health packages evoked frequent opposition because it was making explicit and politically damaging what was already implicit and politically survivable: countries could not pay for everything for everyone. As one policy maker told me *sotto voce* in a southeastern European country in the mid-1990s, it was politically safer to have a delusory constitutional guarantee of comprehensive and free health care if that kept the *lumpenproletariat* happy in their eternal expectations of better days to come, than to address the matter upfront through essential health packages that left some things out.

The 2013 report of The Lancet Commission on Investing in Health includes a concise reflection on criticisms of the 1993 World Development Report. The Commission acknowledged "that user fees can be exclusionary and cause impoverishment, and later in this report we endorse a progressive pathway to UHC that involves zero user fees for poor people."[40]

1.4. Priorities and Players in Practice

Further evolution has placed global health at or close to the forefront of multilateral discourse, with massive political consensus on three concurrent fronts: UHC, development of human capital, and global health security. Whether these define health as an end worth pursuing in and of itself, or as an instrument for economic growth and development, or both, remains a matter of debate in many circles. The World Development Report of 1993 included both. It recognized that good health is an end in itself and that investing in health is a means of improving economic development. As will become clear in later chapters, the onus is on developing countries themselves to make progress toward UHC, despite much rhetoric about global solidarity and despite the performative angst of some Northern NGOs.

The trilogy of priorities — UHC, human capital, and global health security — are situated amidst multiple transitions and threats:

- sociopolitical transition, with greater attention to participatory government and human rights, even as parts of the world fully embrace or flirt with authoritarianism;

- economic transition, as more countries move from low- to middle-income status, but with trajectories now clouded by recessions due to the COVID-19 pandemic;
- governance transition in the post-colonial Global South, both in terms of devolution or decentralization of political, managerial, and administrative authorities in general, and in health in particular, and the slow and uneven development of institutions;
- epidemiologic transition, with chronic noncommunicable diseases becoming more important, even in LICs and MICs, and compounding the unresolved challenges of communicable diseases;[41]
- demographic transition, with parts of the world, especially in many parts of Africa, where poor policy choices with lack of investment in health and education might result in large youthful populations unable to contribute to or benefit from economic growth — putting societies at risk of reaping demographic time bombs instead of demographic dividends;
- climate change;[42]
- pollution;[43,44]
- technological transition, with ever-increasing options in communications, information technology, and biotechnology; and
- transition in the balance of technical expertise, with the Global South increasingly possessing individuals who are the professional and intellectual equals of, and often superior to, would be technical advisors from the Global North, but believing they must accept external policy prescriptions or shoddy technical assistance in order to secure desperately needed funds.

Decades-old global institutions have not always kept pace with these transitions, and none has stayed ahead of the transitions. Traditional purveyors of technical standards struggle for continued primacy, indeed relevance, in a world in which there are more world-class epidemiologists outside than within the WHO, and more such economists outside than within the development banks. The founding charters defined in the immediate aftermath of World War II now appear outdated and attempts by traditional global institutions to justify their existence solely based on mandates put them at risk of irrelevance and functional extinction.

There are legitimate questions about the accountability of powerful foundations and very vocal NGOs of Northern origin that claim to speak on behalf of the underserved and marginalized people of the Global South. Declarations at the United Nations General Assembly, G7, (the short-lived) G8, G20, and other global forums make waves, but their real-life traction is debatable.

The question then arises about the legitimacy and viability, *de jure* and *de facto*, of global health in practice. What and whose narratives shape the practice of global health? From whose policies do the practices arise? By what and whose criteria are successes defined? Is there an unhealthy aversion to recognizing and learning from failures? When well-meaning ambitions such as the United States Global Health Initiative[45] fail, what hope is there for grand alliances on the global stage?[46] Whose reality and interests truly matter during multiparty engagement between the rich Global North and the Global South? These are complex questions with multiple dimensions.

Recent and contemporary literature indicates that many entities and interest groups influence the selection of global health priorities and strategies. While some of that influence comes from financial power, much of it derives from epistemic and normative power, with uncertainties about their legitimacy.[47] But there are equally legitimate questions about the net effects of financial power in global health. When countries of the Global South choose not to pay for their own essential health services, they self-subjugate themselves to others. The resulting dynamics are not those of neo-colonization; they are dynamics of neo-dependency, an acquired disorder that compounds the congenital defects of global imperialism and neo-colonization. These are the discontents now roiling global health.

Imperialism, neo-colonization, and neo-dependency are linked. Their loci of origin might differ, but neo-dependency recapitulates and intensifies the effects of disempowerment wrought by the other two. There are shared qualitative bonds between the invisibility of subjugated people to Sir Alfred Jones, King Leopold II, and Queen Wilhelmina; the invisibility of peoples in much of the contemporary Global South to their own politicians and rulers; the invisibility of Southern institutions and peoples to some Northern purveyors of foreign aid; and the invisibility of Southern peoples to those Northerners who would deny them timely access to technologies to curb the COVID-19 pandemic. The common thread is that the looker chooses not to see the obvious, as in Ralph Ellison's *Invisible Man*:

> *"I am invisible, understand, simply because people refuse to see me. Like the bodiless heads you see sometimes in a circus sideshow, it is as though I have been surrounded by mirrors of hard, distorting glass. When they approach me they see only my surroundings, themselves, or figments of their imagination — indeed, everything and anything except me."*[48]

This book is not a case against foreign aid for health. It is about the dynamics of what works, what does not work, how, and why, in global health. It is about the implicit and explicit discontents in global health investments and opportunities for better performance. It is about what the current system of global health does in practice compared to what it is supposed to do, the reasons for the gaps between exhortations and reality, and plausible changes to optimize for better performance and socio-political legitimacy at the country, regional and global levels. It is about the urgent need to rethink and reform the practice of foreign aid for global health and how it could be done. It is about the debilitating cancer of neo-dependency, of which many politicians and rulers of the Global South seem either enamored or mindlessly accepting. Central to these considerations is a need to check, demystify, and overhaul a massive foreign aid industrial complex, which despite some good intentions and pockets of serious work, often thrives on providing the kind of assistance that the Global South can usefully do without. Equally central is the need to end the culpable neo-dependency that exists in much of the Global South. Whether such changes are best achieved via tinkering with the current practice or overhauling the system is a matter for exploration in the book.

1.5. Structure of the Book

This book is set in nine chapters, including this one. Chapter 2 examines strategic and geopolitical lessons from the COVID-19 pandemic. Beyond the familiar data on disease trends, it zeroes in on a core lesson for the Global South: *in times of severe challenges, you are on your own.* Few lessons are as stark as this amidst the rhetoric of solidarity from the Global North. On this premise, the chapter explores pragmatic options for countries of the Global South as they dig their way out of the disaster of COVID-19 and prepare to do better during future shocks like pandemics. Chapter 3 is the start of a three-chapter package on the challenge of effectively deploying the joint capacities of the public and private sectors for health. It conceptually sets the scene for the following two chapters. Chapter 4, on Malaria Medicines, Markets, and Public Policy, is a first-hand examination of the politics of global health as experienced in the Affordable Medicines Facility-malaria (AMFm), a public–private partnership. Chapter 5 is on Capitalism, Mining, and Restorative Justice in Southern Africa. It explores the industrial roots and current dynamics of health policies, health status, and inequities in the sub-region.

Chapter 6, on the Russian Federation, is the first of two chapters on the dynamics of country realities, government policies, and country engagement with a range of external actors in global health. Chapter 7 is on systemic underperformance and prospects for better health in Nigeria. The chapter zeroes in on abdication of responsibility and poor policy choices as key drivers of underperformance. Chapter 8 is a journey into the real-world dynamics of Development Assistance for Health. It includes composite vignettes — purely for illustrative purposes. Chapter 9, *GPS for Wise Investments in Global Health,* draws lessons from the previous eight chapters and lays out drivers of change for the future.

References

[1] Esteban Ortiz-Ospina and Max Roser. 2016. Health outcomes. In *Global Health.* Published online at OurWorldInData.org. https://ourworldindata.org/health-meta#health-outcomes. Accessed on March 23, 2021.
[2] Hayden J. 2014. The first wealth. https://blogs.imf.org/2014/12/08/the-first-wealth/#:~:text=%E2%80%9CThe%20first%20wealth%20is%20health,%2C%2C%20a%20community%2C%20an%20economy. Accessed on December 15, 2020.

[3] World Health Organization. 2020. Constitution of the World Health Organization. In *Basic Documents: Forty-Ninth Edition* (including amendments adopted up to 31 May 2019). Geneva: World Health Organization. https://apps.who.int/gb/bd/. Accessed on March 23, 2021.

[4] Kipling R. 1899. The white man's burden. https://www.commonlit.org/texts/the-white-man-s-burden. Accessed on May 19, 2021.

[5] Packard RM. 2016. *A History of Global Health*. Baltimore: Johns Hopkins University Press.

[6] Liverpool School of Tropical Medicine. About. https://www.lstmed.ac.uk/history. Accessed on May 19, 2021.

[7] *The London Gazette*. 1901. 27374: 7287, November 9, 1901. https://www.thegazette.co.uk/London/issue/27374/data.pdf. Accessed on May 22, 2021.

[8] Wilkinson L, Power H. 1998. The London and Liverpool schools of tropical medicine 1898–1998. *British Medical Bulletin*, 54(2): 281–292. https://academic.oup.com/bmb/article/54/2/281/284940.

[9] London School of Hygiene and Tropical Medicine. Sir Patrick Manson (1844–1922). https://www.lshtm.ac.uk/aboutus/introducing/history/frieze/sir-patrick-manson. Accessed on July 29, 2021.

[10] Institute of Tropical Medicine Antwerp. Our history. https://www.itg.be/e/-history. Accessed on May 19, 2021.

[11] Hochschild A. 1999. *King Leopold's Ghost. A Story of Greed, Terror, and Heroism in Colonial Africa*. First Mariner Books.

[12] Bishop M, Green M. 2008. *Philanthrocapitalism. How Giving Can Save The World*. New York: Bloomsbury Press.

[13] Giridharadas A. 2018. Winners take all. *The Elite Charade of Changing the World*. New York: Alfred A. Knopf.

[14] KIT Royal Tropical Institute. History. https://www.kit.nl/about-us/history/. Accessed on May 23, 2021.

[15] Shaw C. 2020. Liverpool's slave trade legacy. *History Today*, 70(3). https://www.historytoday.com/history-matters/liverpool's-slave-trade-legacy. Accessed on May 19, 2021.

[16] Lohmann N. 2016. The post colonial transformation of the tropeninstituut: how development aid influenced the direction of the institute from 1945–1979. MA History of International Relations Thesis, University of Amsterdam. p. 47. https://www.kit.nl/wp-content/uploads/2018/10/Thesis-2-1-Niek-Lohmann.pdf. Accessed on May 23, 2021.

[17] Siegal N. 2021. Telling stories of slavery, one person at a time. *New York Times*. https://www.nytimes.com/2021/06/04/arts/design/rijksmuseum-slavery-exhibition.html. Accessed on June 7, 2021.

[18] Writing, theater, arts, and political activism. Conversation with Nobel Laurate Wole Soyinka. Institute of International Studies, University of California, Berkeley. 1998. http://globetrotter.berkeley.edu/conversations/Elberg/Soyinka/soyinka-con4.html. Accessed on June 19, 2021.

[19] Ruger J, 2005 January. The changing role of the World Bank in global health. *American Journal of Public Health,* 95(1): 60–70. https://ajph.aphapublications.org/doi/10.2105/AJPH.2004.042002. Accessed on March 23, 2021.

[20] World Bank. 2021. Universal health coverage. https://www.worldbank.org/en/topic/universalhealthcoverage. Accessed on May 22, 2021.

[21] Bretton Woods Project. 2020. World Bank abandons pandemic bond instrument after disastrous Covid-19 response. https://www.brettonwoodsproject.org/2020/10/world-bank-abandons-pandemic-bond-instrument-after-disastrous-covid-19-response/. Accessed on May 28, 2021.

[22] Nature. 2021. Universal health care must be a priority — even amid COVID. Editorial. *Nature,* 593: 313–314. https://doi.org/10.1038/d41586-021-01313-3. Accessed on May 24, 2021.

[23] Adeyi O, Chopra M, Nandakumar A. 2021. The roads to universal health coverage: manifest destiny or Sisyphean pursuit? Forthcoming. *Journal of Global Health.*

[24] Bryant J. 1969. *Health and the Developing World.* Ithaca, NY: Cornell University Press.

[25] Kickbusch I, Nikogosian H, Kazatchkine M, Kokeny M. 2021. A guide to global health diplomacy. Better health – improved global solidarity – more equity. Graduate Institute of International and Development Studies, Geneva. https://www.graduateinstitute.ch/sites/internet/files/2021-02/GHC-Guide.pdf. Accessed on February 19, 2021.

[26] Kickbush I, Kokeny M. 2013. Global health diplomacy: five years on. *Bulletin of the World Health Organization,* 91:159–159A. https://www.who.int/bulletin/volumes/91/3/13-118596/en/. Accessed on February 19, 2021.

[27] Kopan JP, Bond TC, Merson MH, Reddy KS, Rodriguez MH, Sewankambo NK *et al.* 2009. Towards a common definition of global health. *The Lancet.* https://doi.org/10.1016/S0140-6736(09)60332-9. Accessed on June 6, 2021.

[28] Johns Hopkins Bloomberg School of Public Health. Why we are named the Department of International Health. https://www.jhsph.edu/departments/international-health/about-us/why-the-department-is-named-international-health.html. Accessed on May 19, 2021.

[29] Johns Hopkins University. Center for Global Health. https://hopkinsglobal-health.org. Accessed on June 6, 2021.

[30] Jolly R. Adjustment with a human face: A UNICEF record and perspective on the 1980s. pp. 1807–1921. https://www.sciencedirect.com/science/article/abs/pii/0305750X9190026E. Accessed on December 16, 2020.

[31] Auvinen JY. 1996. IMF intervention and political protest in the third world: A conventional wisdom refined. *Third World Quarterly*, 17(3): 377–400. https://www.jstor.org/stable/3993197?seq=1. Accessed on May 25, 2021.

[32] Fonjong L. 2014. Rethinking the impact of structural adjustment programs on human rights violations in West Africa. *Perspectives on Global Development and Technology*, 13(1–2): 87–110. https://doi.org/10.1163/15691497-12341291. Accessed on May 25, 2021.

[33] Haddad S, Baris E, Narayana D (Eds.). 2008. *Safeguarding the Health System in Times of Macroeconomic Instability. Policy Lessons for Low- and Middle-Income Countries*. Lawrenceville, NJ: Africa World Press.

[34] van der Gaag J, Barhama T. 1998. Health and health expenditures in adjusting and non-adjusting countries. 46(8): 995–1009. https://www.sciencedirect.com/science/article/abs/pii/S0277953697100193?via%3Dihub. Accessed on December 16, 2020.

[35] de Ferranti D. 1985. Paying for health services in developing countries: an overview. World Bank Staff Working Papers. Number 721. http://documents1.worldbank.org/curated/en/485471468739208102/pdf/multi0page.pdf. Accessed on March 23, 2021.

[36] Boseley S. October 2012. From user fees to universal healthcare - a 30-year journey. https://www.theguardian.com/society/sarah-boseley-global-health/2012/oct/01/worldbank-healthinsurance. Accessed on March 23, 2021.

[37] World Bank. 1993. World Development Report 1993. *Investing in Health*. New York: Oxford University Press. https://openknowledge.worldbank.org/handle/10986/5976. Accessed on March 23, 2021.

[38] Lucas A. O. 2010. It was the best of times. *From Local to Global Health*. Ibadan, Nigeria: BookBuilders. p. 275–276.

[39] Bloom D, Canning D, Sevilla. January 2004. The effect of health on economic growth: a production function approach. *World Development*, 32(1): 1–13. https://www.sciencedirect.com/science/article/abs/pii/S0305750X03001943. Accessed on March 23, 2021.

[40] Jamison DT, Summers LH, Alleyne G, Arrow KJ, Berkley S *et al.* 2013. Global health 2035: a world converging within a generation. *The Lancet* (9908): 1898–1955. https://www.thelancet.com/journals/lancet/issue/vol382no9908/PIIS0140-6736(13)X6061-1. Accessed on June 9, 2021.

[41] Adeyi O, Smith O, Robles S. 2007. Public policy and the challenge of chronic noncommunicable diseases. Directions in Development. Human Development. Washington, DC: World Bank. https://openknowledge.worldbank.org/handle/10986/6761. Accessed on March 23, 2021.

[42] Watts N, Amann M, Arnell N, Karlsson S, Beagley J, Belesova K *et al.* 2020. The 2020 report of the *Lancet* countdown on health and climate change: responding to converging crises. *The Lancet*, 397(10269):129–170. https://doi.org/10.1016/S0140-6736(20)32290-X. Accessed on March 23, 2021.

[43] Preker AS, Adeyi OO, Lapetra MG, Simon D, Keuffel E. 2017. Health care expenditures associated with pollution: exploratory methods and findings. *Annuals of Global Health*, 82(5): 711–721. http://doi.org/10.1016/j.aogh.2016.12.003. Accessed on March 23, 2021.

[44] Landrigan P, Fuller R, Acosta N, Adeyi O, Arnold R, Basu N *et al.* 2017. The Lancet Commission on pollution and health. *The Lancet*. Published online on October 19, 2017. https://www.thelancet.com/pdfs/journals/lancet/PIIS0140-6736(17)32345-0.pdf Accessed on March 23, 2021.

[45] Alcorn T. 2012. What has the US global health initiative achieved? *The Lancet*. 380(9849):1216–1216. https://www.thelancet.com/journals/lancet/article/PIIS0140-6736(12)61697-3/fulltext. Accessed on May 5, 2021.

[46] Pai M. 2019. Archives of failures in global health. *Nature Microbiology Community*. http://naturemicrobiologycommunity.nature.com/posts/51659-archive-of-failures-in-global-health. Accessed on May 5, 2021.

[47] Shiffman J. Knowledge, moral claims and the exercise of power in global health. https://www.ijhpm.com/article_2918.html.

[48] Ellison, R. 1995. *Invisible Man*. New York: Vintage Books. 1995 Edition.

Chapter 2

Strategic and Geopolitical Lessons from COVID-19

"Predicting rain doesn't count; building arks does."

—Warren Buffett[a]

*"At a more general level, conflicts between the rich and poor are
unlikely because, except in special circumstances, the poor countries
lack the political unity, economic power, and military capability to challenge the rich countries. Rich states may fight trade wars with each
other; poor states may fight violent wars with each other; but an international class war between the poor South and wealthy North is almost
as far from reality as one happy harmonious world."*

—Samuel Huntington[b]

Synopsis

The COVID-19 pandemic has concentrated minds on the fact that contrary
to everyday assumptions, humans are not the boss species on earth.
A virus, invisible to the naked eye, can inflict severe damage on lives and

[a]Berkshire Hathaway Inc. 2001. Annual Report. p. 9. https://www.berkshirehathaway.com/2001ar/2001ar.pdf.
[b]Huntington SP. 1996. *The Clash of Civilizations and the Remaking of World Order.* New York: Simon & Schuster. p. 33.

livelihoods, bring economies to their knees, remove the veneers of civility within countries, and amplify grudges and hostilities among nations. Crucially, the stark inequities between the Global North and the Global South, combined with COVID nationalism around medical equipment and vaccines, sent a clear message to countries of the Global South: in moments of great peril, they cannot count on the rich countries of the Global North for timely solidarity. It is now clear that the International Health Regulations (IHR) rested on unfounded assumptions that norms and platitudes of solidarity would triumph over incentives and national self-interests. What stands between country populations and absolute disasters is the resilience of their institutions amidst stress. With health now more broadly understood as a matter of national security and a bedrock of global security, the production and distribution of strategic medical equipment, drugs, and vaccines is too important to be left to the market alone. Governments should strategically and selectively invest in industrial production and supply chains. It is past time for the Global South to take responsibility for its own future and leave behind its dependency on the Global North.

2.1. The Sum of All Threats

The COVID-19 pandemic is the convergence of multiple threats. On January 30, 2020, WHO declared the outbreak of the SARS-CoV-2 virus a public health emergency of international concern (PHEIC). That is WHO's highest level of alert.[1] By July 29, 2021, WHO had received reports of 195,886,929 confirmed cases of COVID-19, including 4,189,148 deaths.[2] It will take years to fully understand and document the vast ramifications of COVID-19.[3,4] However, the first year of the pandemic has shown that the very technocratic country rankings from the Global Health Security Index[5] were not predictive of effective responses to pandemics. This was true of some of the highest-ranked countries like the United States and United Kingdom, whose responses during 2020 showed how dysfunctional political leadership could undermine the effectiveness of otherwise strong technical institutions. Jamison and others recently showed the potential of "objectively generated measures of country performance" to inform the evaluation of policy choices and enhance the accountability of policy makers.[6]

It is already clear that the COVID-19 pandemic is the sum of multiple threats, prominent among which are the following seven:

(1) The first threat is biological and environmental. Regardless of the ultimate finding on the immediate origin of the virus — whether from a marketplace, or a laboratory, or an unknown index case in some forest — humanity remains at risk of other outbreaks, any of which could be even more infectious, more pathogenic, and more lethal.

(2) The second threat is political. Especially in the first year of the pandemic, the world saw in real time the ramifications and disastrous consequences of executive incompetence across country income levels.[7,8] During 2020, concurrent with COVID-19 leadership failures in the United States,[9] the United Kingdom,[10] Brazil,[11–13] and Tanzania,[14] there were examples of effective leadership across income levels in New Zealand, Vietnam, and Taiwan, among others. Despite prior warnings of the danger of false optimism in 2020,[15] the devastating second waves of COVID-19 in India in April and May 2021 appeared to have resulted from a combination of leadership failure, an unscientific response to the pandemic, and complacency,[16–18] with implications for the rest of the world.[19]

(3) The third threat is social; in times of sudden and then prolonged stress, the veneer of civility can be very thin, with individual behaviors ranging from an ethos of "I will do my part and contribute to the solution" to an ethos of "my right to inflict damage on others knows no bounds."

(4) The fourth threat is that of dysfunctional systems of production and supply chains for mission-critical equipment and supplies, including diagnostic and therapeutic machinery and consumables, medicines, and vaccines. They buckled under stress and collapsed in many places. That realization has prompted attention to and reviews of the security of medical product supply chains, including in the United States.[20,21]

(5) The fifth threat arises from the absence, weakness, or dysfunction of institutions for epidemiological surveillance, outbreak detection, and effective response to disease outbreaks.

(6) The sixth threat arises from combinations of economic collapse and inability to mount sufficiently strong short-term responses to cushion the shocks caused by disruptions of commercial activities within and across countries.

(7) The seventh threat is a combination of vaccine nationalism, geopolitical brinkmanship, and bickering, which condemns most countries to prolonged waits for solutions.

The rest of this chapter highlights the strategic and geopolitical lessons arising from the global exposure to these threats. It is an intra-pandemic perspective that could evolve as more is learned about the dynamics and sequelae of the pandemic. These lessons are grounded in the premise that while pandemic preparedness and response have crucial technical and institutional dimensions, the strategic and geopolitical dimensions are foundational and have multiplier effects that shape all other dimensions.

2.2. Message from the Global North: You Are on Your Own

COVID-19 is an existential threat to humans across the world and a serious threat to economies. It makes sense to cooperate in a fight against a common enemy, especially when that enemy is a virus that constitutes an existential threat. Models indicate that strategies based on cooperation are more effective in containing pandemics when supplies of antivirals are limited and reproductive rates approach 1.9. These findings apply across the world and hold for countries that share their resources with others.[22,23] But the reality in the COVID-19 pandemic is a breakdown between the countries that manufacture essential equipment and those that buy such equipment but don't make them.

In the first year of the pandemic, that breakdown featured a scramble for medical equipment — especially respirators and personal protective equipment such as face masks, breakdown of supply chains because of insufficient production, disrupted production, breakdowns of global and regional air transport corridors, border closures, and hoarding of goods and supplies. The breakdowns across product categories, which have since extended to vaccines, have classic features of a tragedy of the commons.[24] In plain speak, the message from the Global North to the Global South could not be clearer: *you are on your own during times of great peril.*

It is not the case that the Global North has pursued its own narrow interests at the margins of the common interest, in so far as the common interest is defined by equity-based mechanisms led or brokered by multilateral entities such as the WHO, Gavi, and CEPI in collaboration with country leaders. The reality amidst a severe pandemic, which by definition is a global problem, is that the Global North set out to pursue its own narrow interests as the main event, and those multilateral mechanisms are side-shows to be tolerated, acknowledged, and used for public relations props. The poster child for that marginalization is the ACT Accelerator:[25]

> *"The Access to COVID-19 Tools (ACT) Accelerator, is a groundbreaking global collaboration to accelerate development, production, and equitable access to COVID-19 tests, treatments, and vaccines.*
>
> *Launched at the end of April 2020, at an event co-hosted by the Director-General of the World Health Organization, the President of France, the President of the European Commission, and the Bill & Melinda Gates Foundation, the Access to COVID-19 Tools (ACT) Accelerator brings together governments, scientists, businesses, civil society, and philanthropists and global health organizations (the Bill & Melinda Gates Foundation, CEPI, FIND, Gavi, The Global Fund to Fight AIDS, Tuberculosis and Malaria, Unitaid, Wellcome, the WHO, and the World Bank).*
>
> *The ACT-Accelerator is organized into four pillars of work: diagnostics, treatment, vaccines and health system strengthening. Each pillar is vital to the overall effort and involves innovation and collaboration. Cross-cutting all of the work, and fundamental to the goals of the ACT-Accelerator, is the Access and Allocation workstream that is led by WHO and is developing the principles, framework and mechanisms needed to ensure the fair and equitable allocation of these tools."*

COVAX, the vaccines component of the Access to COVID-19 Tools (ACT) Accelerator, included the following among its self-declared goals: (i) doses for at least 20% of country populations; (ii) an actively managed portfolio of diverse vaccines; (iii) prompt delivery of available vaccines; (iv) bring to an end the acute phase of the pandemic; and (v) economic recovery. For all public relations purposes, it was aimed at the Global South.[26]

The modest goal of COVAX — essentially pegged at 20% coverage — is incongruent with the lofty objectives of curbing COVID-19 as a public health disaster *and* rebuilding economies. WHO notes that the level of vaccine coverage needed for herd immunity to COVID-19 is unknown. Furthermore, there are variations across diseases in the percentage of the population who must be immune in order to reach herd immunity. The percentage is about 95% for measles and about 80% for poliomyelitis.[27] If curbing COVID-19 is a pre-requisite for getting back to the normal functions of societies and economies, even 20% coverage with vaccines will not do because that level of vaccine coverage falls far short of what would plausibly give vaccine-induced herd immunity to SARS-CoV-2.[28] The Global North would never accept COVAX as the definitive solution for its own population, based on those same targets.

It is hard to conclude that COVAX was engineered to be the common pathway to *a definitive and robust solution* for the Global South. From early stages, even the modest goals were being threatened as wealthy countries bilaterally entered into separate purchase contracts with manufactures of COVID-19 vaccines, creating a *de facto* hoard for rich countries only. These bilateral deals effectively hobbled COVAX because COVAX did not have the funds to compete with wealthy countries that cornered the market from the beginning by striking purchase deals with vaccine manufacturers.[29] The behavior of Canada is an example of how the Global North undermined the response to COVID-19. On the one hand, Canada has been a major financial contributor to COVAX. On the other hand, Canada and other rich countries subverted COVAX through bilateral deals with vaccine suppliers, thereby pushing COVAX toward the back of the line for scarce global supplies.[30,31]

Since it was impossible for poorer countries and institutions like Gavi and WHO (both of which depend on funds from the rich countries) to stop those bilateral deals, some have suggested options based on a game-theory perspective to structure those bilateral deals in ways that could improve the global supply of vaccines.[32] The real-life COVAX experience is close to what wise poker players learn very early: it is essential to identify the patsy at the table — and doubly important to do so early in the game. Anyone who fails to do so is likely to be the patsy. LICs and MICs of the Global South approached the COVID-19 response as if it were a mutual support movement, only to realize that the rich countries of the Global North were playing them for suckers in a high-stakes geopolitical cold war.

2.3. Feast for the West, Famine for the Rest

"The 5.6 billion people who don't live in the West deeply resent the presumption that 900 million westerners should be calling the global shots politically and economically."

—Matt Miller[c]

Figure 2.1. shows, by region, the share of populations who had gotten at least one dose of a COVID-19 vaccine as of early May 2021.

The reality as of the third quarter of 2021 was that the Global North was parochially pursuing the protection of its own population in a quest for vaccine-induced herd immunity. Concurrently, the Global North had adopted a trickle-down approach to the Global South. Vaccines would be donated or provided to the Global South if and when there were surpluses in the Global North, where rich countries have purchased most of the existing vaccine supplies as of early 2021. The hoarding of vaccines by countries such as Canada[33] and the United States,[34,35] the internecine vitriol among the European Union countries and the United Kingdom,[36,37] approaching the Global South as a theater of a cold war over vaccines,[38,39] and the cringeworthy celebration of greed[40] point to the power of unbridled short-term self-interests over the collective good. The randomness of nationality or country of residence, indeed, determines people's chances of survival.[41] There are reasons to conclude that the political economy of

---

[c]Miller M. 2009. *The Tyranny of Dead Ideas*. New York: Times Books. p. 149.

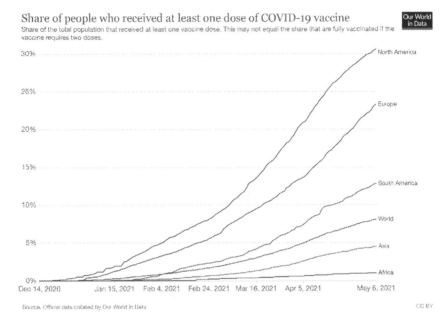

Figure 2.1.   Share of People Who Received at Least One Dose of COVID-19 Vaccine

COVID-19 has revealed pre-existing dynamics of resource extraction and its association with imperialism and racism.[42]

Yet, despite the stance of the rich Global North, it is benefiting from the generosity of the poor Global South. Hard-hit Italy, a member of the European Union, received aid from Cuba in its fight against COVID-19.[43]

> *"In Lombardy ... everyone is grateful for their professionalism and their humbleness and availability to a country they hardly know," said Marco Grimaldi, a politician from north-west Italy who helped to negotiate the arrival of a group of 39 Cuban healthcare workers with diplomats from Havana. "Imagine if Europe could manage to do the same."*

These actions are taking place in a context of severe economic effects of the pandemic, which the LICs and MICs are less well placed to mitigate compared to the HICs. The IMF has reported that access to financing has shaped fiscal responses: average overall deficits as a share of GDP in 2020 were projected at –13.3% for advanced economies, –10.3% for emerging market and middle-income economies, and –5.7% for low-income developing countries. More specifically, the IMF reported unprecedented fiscal expansion for advanced economies, differentiated fiscal responses for emerging markets and MICs, and modest fiscal support for the LICs.[44] Remarkably, the IMF noted in the same report the importance of global solidarity to ensure access to vaccines and treatments. In July 2021, the IMF's economic growth forecast portrayed a divergence between the vaccine-rich Global North and the vaccine-deprived Global South. With almost 40% of their populations fully vaccinated, 2021 growth projections for advanced economies had improved by 0.5%. That increase was offset exactly by a downward revision for emerging markets (with 11% of their populations fully vaccinated) and developing economies (with only a tiny fraction of their populations fully vaccinated). For 2022, the IMF projected an appreciable upgrade for advanced economies and a more modest increase for emerging market and developing economies.[45]

The inescapable conclusion is stark: LICs and LMICs are fighting COVID-19 with both arms tied behind their backs because they lack the fiscal firepower of the Global North and they lack access to vaccines, a situation that is hampered by multiple dimensions of vaccine hoarding by the Global North. In addition, the emergency repurposing of staff and equipment from routine health care delivery to COVID-19 services is likely to cause more preventable illnesses and premature deaths in LICs and MICs.

2.4. Not Sapiens: Paralysis and Obfuscation at WTO's TRIPS Council

Amidst a pandemic that has exposed many systemic inadequacies, it makes sense to deploy comprehensive measures to ensure that everyone has timely and equitable access to vaccines, diagnostics, and therapeutics. Waiving intellectual property (IP) rights that constrain a broader base for manufacturing vaccines is important, even if doing so will not instantaneously increase vaccine production in the Global South. It is crucial that the Global North and the Global South sensibly — and urgently — resolve the question of intellectual property rights to certain medical tools and technologies. Yet, entrenched interests in the Global North have acted as if these were normal times. In 2020, South Africa and India asked the World Trade Organization (WTO) to suspend intellectual property (IP) rights related to COVID-19. The rationale was to vastly expand access to affordable COVID-related medicines, vaccines, and other mission-critical technologies beyond the HICs. Many LICs and MICs supported the call. The patent waiver proposal was presented to the WTO's Trade-Related Aspects of Intellectual Property (TRIPS) Council on October 16, 2020 and discussed again at a council meeting on November 20, 2020.[46]

Proponents argued that a waiver would make it possible for manufacturers and governments to speed up vaccine supply. That is a different scenario from an exclusively charity-based approach in which HICs would dole out inadequate quantities of vaccines that are surplus to their own domestic requirement when they so pleased. Many HICs objected to the request for a waiver, claiming that it would undermine innovation. The initial objections came from the European Union, the United Kingdom, the United States, and most of the larger pharmaceutical firms. They argued that such waivers were both unnecessary and undesirable for COVID-19 vaccines.[47,48]

In an indication of the commitment to blocking the proposal, the pharmaceutical industry's pushback included a letter from the Pharmaceutical Research and Manufacturers of America (PhRMA) to United States President Joseph Biden.[49] Their argument that an IP waiver would undermine incentives to finance innovation does not pass scrutiny. The assumption that patents create positive incentives for innovation is common, but it is highly contested in academic scholarship.[50] Besides, big pharmaceutical companies rely on and benefit from public money that funds basic research. In the United States alone, six vaccines reportedly have received about US$12 billion of public funds, and public funds reportedly paid about 97% of the development costs of the AstraZeneca/ Oxford vaccine. Prior publicly funded research benefits vaccine development.[51] Thus did these pharmaceutical companies seek to socialize costs and privatize benefits behind the monopoly-granting regime of IP at the WTO.

The South African Government responded to objections, pointing to examples of how IP has created barriers to access. Of particular note is India's statement to the November 20, 2019 TRIPS Council:

> *"On one hand, these countries are buying up as much of the limited supply as they can, leaving no vaccines in the pie for developing and least-developed countries. On the other hand, and very strangely, these are the same countries who are arguing against the need for the waiver that can help increase the global manufacturing and supply to achieve not just equitable, but also timely and affordable access to such vaccines for all countries."*[46]

It is true that the suspension of IP rights *alone* will not, *in the short run*, resolve the supply shortage of COVID-19 vaccines. This is because of the high costs and technical complexities of vaccine development and manufacturing. Those challenges are compounded by shortages of key inputs into manufacturing, which is a problem even for established vaccine manufacturers in the Global South. Yadav and Weintraub succinctly laid out four pathways to increase the global supply of COVID-19 vaccines: improve the flow of the raw materials; harmonize regulatory processes; expand vaccine-manufacturing capacity; and establish a supply chain informatory.[52] Jha and colleagues outlined an integrated three-pillar global vaccine compact to expand vaccine supply and counter vaccine nationalism: country adult vaccination programs based on the idea of a fully immunized adult; a global vaccine manufacturing compact housed in less populous countries with good scientific and training infrastructure, a respect for legal contracts, and a reputation for fair play; and rapidly expanding production capacity by private pharmaceutical companies without encouraging the rent-seeking behavior enabled by patent law.[53] These proposals make sense, and the authors noted that the highly successful (but unfortunately defunct) Affordable Medicines Facility for malaria (AMFm) has already shown how to constructively engage with the private sector. The AMFm is examined in detail in Chapter 4.

It is also true that suspending IP rights does not preclude those strategies; it is an essential part of a comprehensive and robust strategy. However, by mid-2021, at least 10 meetings in 7 months had failed to move WTO members toward consensus on the original waiver proposal.[54]

Only after coming under intense pressure did the administration of President Joseph Biden agree to lift restrictions on exports of supplies that vaccine makers in India said they needed to expand production amid a devastating surge in COVID-19 deaths there.[55,56] It took more pressure for the Biden Administration to announce its support for the waiver.[57] In a swift and quasi-apocalyptic objection to that support, the International Federation of Pharmaceutical Manufacturers and Associations (IFPMA) failed to credibly explain why the TRIPS waiver and the measures outlined by IFPMA had to be mutually exclusive:[58]

> *"We are fully aligned with the goal to ensure COVID-19 vaccines are quickly and equitably shared around the world. But, as we have consistently stated, a waiver is the simple but the wrong answer to what is a complex problem. Waiving patents of COVID-19 vaccines will not increase production nor provide practical solutions needed to battle this global health crisis. On the contrary, it is likely to lead to disruption; while distracting from addressing the real challenges in scaling up production and distribution of COVID-19 vaccines globally: namely elimination of trade barriers, addressing bottlenecks in supply chains and scarcity of raw materials and ingredients in the supply chain, and a willingness by rich countries to start sharing doses with poor countries."*

Faced with a shift in the American position, European governments offered an incoherent mix of responses, ranging from the European Commission's position that "the EU is also ready to discuss any proposals that address the crisis in an effective and pragmatic manner" (after having declared a few weeks earlier that it did not favor IP waivers[59]), to France's statement that it was "absolutely in favor" (a marked shift in stance for France, which had earlier taken the position that IP waivers would undermine innovation[60]), to the statement from an unnamed United Kingdom government spokesperson that his country was "working with WTO members to resolve this issue" and was "in discussions with the US and WTO members to facilitate increased production and supply of COVID-19 vaccines".[61,62] France then equivocated, wondering whether it was really about intellectual property, and asserting that "the Anglo-Saxons block many of these ingredients and vaccines."[63] Thus, while sending naval boats to confront post-Brexit Britain,[64] did France find a brilliant solution to the problem of vaccine apartheid: it retreated to its visceral comfort zone of lambasting both the Perfidious Albion across the English Channel and the Hyperpower across the Atlantic. Never mind the last two words in "Liberté, égalité, fraternité," the people of the Global South were expendable.

There is a geopolitical straight line from the ruinous indemnity debt that France imposed on freedom-seeking Haiti in the 19th Century to its placement of IP rights held by companies of the Global North above the human rights of the Global South to health, this time via vaccines.[65] The logic is the same: if the Global South wants freedom from the bondage of IP on COVID-19 vaccines and other medical technologies amidst the existential threat of a pandemic, it should pay crippling royalties, despite the fact that the Global North benefits from data on SARS-CoV-2 genome sequencing performed by scientists all over the world, including the Global South.[66] The waffling by the United Kingdom government indicates that the "wealth" in The Commonwealth is common only when it flows from the former colonies to Westminster.

Let us now reflect on the case of Germany and its opposition to the waiver of IP rights as of mid-2021. In 1989, the world rejoiced with Berliners as the city was reunified after decades of externally imposed division that followed World War II. Cheering the good fortune of others is the right thing to do. But lost in that outpouring of goodwill was Berlin's record as the city where the fates of other people were sealed through externally imposed divisions: the General Act of Berlin on The Scramble for Africa was signed there in 1885,[67] and there followed dire consequences for others.[68] Germany, whose West Berlin benefited from the extraordinary Berlin Airlift in 1948–1949 when it was blockaded by the Soviet Union,[69] and which benefited from the generosity of spirit in President John F. Kennedy's *"Ich bin ein Berliner!"* speech,[70] swiftly rejected the United States-backed proposal to waive IP rights on COVID-19 vaccines.[61]

By opposing the waiver of IP rights on COVID-19 vaccines, the German government indirectly denies billions of people the opportunity that people in Germany have, that of vaccination against COVID-19. That is the sobering reality. Among the hundreds of millions of people from whom Germany would have pharmaceutical companies extort IP royalties for COVID-19 vaccines are descendants of those whose societies were devastated by the consequences of the General Act of Berlin on The Scramble for Africa. They include the Herero, about 75% of whose forebears perished in Germany's state-mandated massacre in German South-West Africa, the modern-day Namibia. In matters of danger to lives and livelihoods across the world, an insistence on looking out for oneself alone and opposition to equitable global solutions is a geopolitical act of selfishness and, arguably, *schadenfreude*. A solidarity-based stance that rose to the occasion would be *"Ich bin ein Weltbürger!"*[d]

During the 20th century, Europe twice globalized its domestic tribal wars and exploited the peoples and treasures of its colonies to fight for freedom in Europe while denying those colonies the same freedoms. Much of the wealth of Europe was built on the plunder of peoples and goods from the subjugated colonies. Many European countries continue to keep in their museums priceless intellectual property in the form of artworks that Europeans looted from the colonies. Yet, when there is a dire global threat to health and economies, and those former colonies need solidarity, European governments have been models of isolationism, selfishness, and charity-based tokenism. The behavior of European governments exemplified injustices[71] that should be eliminated from global health. On July 27, 2021, the European Commission released a statement that epitomized both parochial triumphalism and geopolitical tone-deafness (Box 2.1). It came amidst a devastating surge of the Delta variant of SARS-CoV-2 across the Global South, where only a tiny fraction of the population had been vaccinated. It accompanied EU vaccine nationalism and opposition to IP waivers. On display was a policy of feasting the West while starving the rest. The African Union wanted to buy vaccines but vaccine-hoarding Europe and North America preferred the cynical tokenism of measly donations to Africa. Sometimes, those donated vaccines were close to expiry.

---

[d]A nonnative speaker's attempt at "I am a citizen of the world."

Box 2.1. Europe's Vaccine Nationalism and Selfishness

Statement by President von der Leyen on a new milestone in the EU Vaccines Strategy.

The EU has kept its word and delivered.

Our target was to protect 70% of adults in the European Union with at least one vaccination in July.

Today we have achieved this target. And 57% of adults already have the full protection of double vaccination.

These figures put Europe among the world leaders.

The catch-up process has been very successful — but we need to keep up the effort.

The delta variant is very dangerous. I therefore call on everyone — who has the opportunity — to be vaccinated. For their own health and to protect others.

The EU will continue to provide sufficient volumes of vaccine.

Source: European Commission. 2021. https://ec.europa.eu/commission/presscorner/detail/en/STATEMENT_21_3921. Accessed on July 27, 2021.

The observed behaviors of European governments and leaders raises a question. When European political leaders claim leadership in global health,[72,73] are they being genuine, or do they merely seek photo opportunities to boost their images by standing next to little brown children from the Global South while ruthlessly denying the families of those children access to life-saving technologies like COVID-19 vaccines?

The failure of the Global North to rise to the occasion is not uniquely European. While the Presidency of the European Commission was gloating despite a global imbalance, the United States was on the verge of wasting millions of doses of the COVID-19 vaccines that were close to expiring. That was after hoarding the vaccines for months,[74] a fact that cannot be erased by highly publicized token donations to countries of the Global South. During the same week, *Nature* published a *cri-de-coeur* by a Liberia-based author who drew attention to the fact that "rich countries are hoarding vaccines, allowing doses to expire while unvaccinated people who want to be immunized die."[75] The COVID-19 pandemic held a mirror to humanity and the reflection in the mirror was neither pretty nor noble.

The strategic and geopolitical issues are bigger than the very real short-term technical constraints on vaccine manufacturing in the Global South. If an appropriate vow in the wake of COVID-19 is that never again will humanity be so unprepared and at loggerheads over how to confront a shared threat, it behooves the Global North to invest in both short-term and medium-term global solutions, not just for its own population, and not only on its own geographic territories. If countries of the Global South truly stand no chance of manufacturing vaccines if IP rights related to COVID-19 were suspended, what are the entrenched hegemonic interests of the Global North so afraid of? There is a fear of losing geopolitical advantages to China,[76,77] which "has become the foremost practitioner in the world of geo-economics — the use of economic instruments of power to achieve unrelated political and strategic objectives even as it pursues its economic interests."[78] That consideration, it appears, outweighs the lives of billions of people in the Global South, who are supposed to line up as pawns in yet another cold war.

Leaders of the Global South would be well advised to take a two-pronged approach. The first is to recognize that despite the unhelpful political positions taken by several of the G7 governments and politicians, there are many constituencies of enduring goodwill in the G7 countries, and those constituencies believe in equitable access to life-saving technologies to fight the pandemic. This realization provides reasons to continue seeking common grounds in the interest of bringing the pandemic under control. The second is to concurrently chart their own paths out of the pandemic, form transparent and nonexploitative alliances with whomever can meaningfully help achieve their goals, and heed the injunction of Nelson Mandela:[79]

> "One of the mistakes that the outside world makes is to think that their enemies should be our enemies. Our attitude toward any country is determined by the attitude of that country toward our struggle."
>
> "We are not looking at any particular model. As far as economic policy is concerned, our sole concern is that the inequalities which are to be found in the economy should be redressed."

Some influential institutions in the Global North have built up a false narrative about the proposition for a TRIPs waiver regarding technologies that are essential for curbing the pandemic. For example, the *Washington Post*'s Editorial Board ran the following on May 3, 2021:[80]

> *"It is true that pharmaceutical companies stand to profit handsomely from monopolies on individual patented vaccines. It is also true that stripping away their intellectual property now could discourage future innovation. The U.S. government spent some $10 billion in Operation Warp Speed to help that effort, among other things, but did not require companies to turn over their intellectual property to the government — or to share it."*

The *Washington Post*'s Editorial Board's position is at odds with the fact that the swift development of COVID-19 vaccines benefited from publicly funded basic research conducted by scientists at federal institutions.[81] In addition, it was revealingly uncritical of billions of taxpayers' money being spent to confer monopolistic profits on commercial entities. Given the propensity of many large companies for rigging the tax code in their favor by lobbying the United States Congress,[82] it is entirely possible that the government gets not one dime of the stream of profits. If this happened in the Global South, the *Washington Post* might excoriate it as crony capitalism. But it gets worse in the same editorial:

> *"The most salient fact is that patents on vaccines are not the central bottleneck, and even if turned over to other nations, would not quickly result in more shots. This is because vaccine manufacturing is exacting and time-consuming. Look at the production difficulties encountered by Emergent BioSolutions, a vaccine manufacturer in Baltimore, where 15 million doses were contaminated. That was caught before the shots were distributed, but one can imagine the horrific consequences of a failure to maintain quality control elsewhere in the world."*

As noted earlier, merely waiving IP rights will not solve the problem of COVID-19 vaccine shortage in the short run. But the *Washington Post*'s own logic would lead to some unintended consequences. For example, should the production of vaccines be suspended in the Global North because they are demonstrably incapable of producing vaccines without contamination in Baltimore,[83,84] which is only 40 miles from the *Washington Post* headquarters? Because of that blunder in Baltimore, Emergent BioSolutions could not deliver millions of doses of Johnson & Johnson's COVID-19 vaccines to Canada, Europe, and South Africa. By the same logic, should the infrastructure plan of the Biden Administration[85] be stopped because of the horrific failures of the "big dig" in Boston?[86] The *Washington Post* invented what it could imagine as the basis for its specious argument, and projected that imagination onto the Global South. Some due diligence and global situation awareness would have alerted the *Washington Post* to relevant facts. India, one of the world's largest vaccine manufacturers, is not located in North America, but is part of that "elsewhere in the world." There are opportunities on which to build a vaccine development infrastructure in Africa.[87,88]

The *Washington Post*'s Editorial Board then outdid itself in another editorial, which concluded with the following:[89]

> *"The second effort over the longer term is for the United States, Europe and others to help boost vaccine supply, manufacturing capacity and raw materials for these hard-hit nations. Start by donating surplus shots. Beyond the valuable Covax initiative now underway, wealthy nations should lend experienced personnel and manufacturing know-how to produce vaccines at scale and on the ground, which is far more useful than lifting patent protection. Why not create an Operation Global Vax to rush this vital aid to developing nations with the same urgency and ambition as Operation Warp Speed in the United States? Let's give them what they genuinely need."*

In calling for an "Operation Global Vax," the *Washington Post*'s Editorial Board paid no heed to the steps that wealthy nations of the Global North took to hobble COVAX; it was time to move on to some shiny new charity operation without an honest appraisal of COVAX. But that manifestation of attention deficit disorder was not the geopolitical sleight of hand at play here. It was the last sentence of the editorial that was revealing as a dog whistle in the geopolitics of DAH: an entity in the Global North implicitly or explicitly assumed divine rights and omniscience (on behalf of some "we" or "us") to determine what the Global South ("them" or "they") needed, and either ignored or rode roughshod over whatever the Global South itself specified that it needed. The basis on which the *Washington Post* decided which needs were genuine and which were not is unknown, but it sought to rubbish in a single stroke the case led by India and South Africa at the WTO. It is reminiscent of the approach taken by many political leaders of the Global North when they refused to impose sanctions on the apartheid regime in South Africa: they presumed to know better than those representing the victims of apartheid. Then and now, it was a ploy to preserve the *status quo* that unjustly favored short-term commercial interests of the Global North.

The weekly journal *Nature*, unlike the *Washington Post*, understood both the fundamental issues at stake and the moral importance of being on the right side of history. It noted European pledges to increase vaccine donations to countries of the Global South made at the Global Health Summit in Rome[90] and at the World Health Assembly in Geneva, both in May 2021. In its editorial, entitled "A patent waiver on COVID vaccines is right and fair," *Nature* then delivered this comment for the ages:[91]

> *"These commitments are crucial in the race to end the pandemic. But they do not deal with the systemic issue — countries backing the IP waiver are not asking for charity, but for the right to develop and make their own vaccines, free from the worry that they will be sued by patent holders. Those backing the COVID IP waiver understand this core principle. The leaders of countries that are not currently in favor of the patent waiver must recognize it, too."*

That *Nature* editorial should be required reading for every delegate to every forum on global health. It is at the core of geopolitical influences on the response to the COVID-19 pandemic.

The World Bank's opposition to IP waivers for COVID-19 vaccines was a craven abdication of the duty of care in curbing disease and poverty. Asked about the proposal for waiving COVID-19 vaccine IP, World Bank President David Malpass reportedly said: "We don't support that, for the reason that it would run the risk of reducing the innovation and the R&D in that sector."[92] That position is not helpful to the millions of poor people in the Global South whose lives and livelihoods are being ravaged by COVID-19. It puts purportedly long-term gains of vaccine innovation (spurred by IP rights that allow patent holders to monopolize the benefits of largely government-funded research) above the compelling short- to medium-term need to expand access to COVID-19 vaccines.

The anti-IP waiver position taken by the *Washington Post* and the World Bank, among others, strengthens the hands of the already powerful pharmaceutical industry lobby. It also muddies the waters to the disadvantage of the Global South. For example, the position confers an illusion of great progress on the tokenism of Pfizer and BioNTech's announcement in July 2021 of an agreement with a South African manufacturer to perform the final steps of manufacturing and distributing their vaccine in Africa. It was only the fill-and-finish phase of manufacturing, but the breathless hype around it was almost as if Pfizer and BioNTech were going to waive the IP for that vaccine and engage in deep technology transfer with the sharing of know-now across the value chain, which is what they should be doing in the face of a devastating pandemic. Global health tokenism was publicized as a fundamental shift.

Given the severity of the COVID-19 emergency, it is a political, ethical, and moral failure to not waive those IP rights. Potential resolutions that fall short of suspending IP rights to COVID-related medical products include elements of nonexclusive licenses and technology transfer of patented products. Confining an agreement to voluntary licensing alone is not a robust solution in a world divided into the haves of the Global North and the have-nots of the Global South. It is the vaccine supply equivalent of trickle-down economics: the rich gain at the expense of the poor.[92]

The world is at an impasse. The revealed stance of the Global North is: *what is yours is ours and what is mine is mine*. The Global North is running a long-term risk and it might rue its current posture when the Global South acquires both the technology and sufficient economic might to turn the tables. One could imagine a situation in which countries of the Global South adopt a variation of the decision by Indonesia to withhold samples of avian influenza virus A (H5N1) from the WHO in 2007,[93] and combine that policy with technological prowess. It is hard to imagine the Global North demonstrating philosophical calm and agreeing with that stance, or suddenly discovering fairness in a stance that trivializes an existential threat to the health of its own population. This is what makes the current stance of the Global North contrary to its own long-run interests.

If aliens from another galaxy were to assess humanity's collective response to COVID-19 as of mid-2021, they would declare it a failure because humanity has not lived up to the *sapiens* label. The Report of the Independent Panel on Pandemic Preparedness and Response, which contains very insightful and potentially high-impact recommendations, still falls short of the boldness required to outgrow the ossified *status quo*. It sensibly seeks to: put pandemic preparedness and response at the highest level of political leadership; strengthen the independence, authority, and financing of WHO; invest in preparedness to prevent the next crisis; introduce an agile and rapid surveillance information and alert system; establish a prenegotiated platform for tools and supplies; raise new international financing for pandemic preparedness and response; and empower National Pandemic coordinators with direct lines to Heads of State or Government. However, all these would take place within the current power dynamics between the Global North and the Global South. In a revealing signal of how hobbled the Panel was, it made the following call:[94]

> *"The World Trade Organization (WTO) and WHO should convene major vaccine-producing countries and manufacturers to agree to voluntary licensing and technology transfer for COVID-19 vaccines. If actions do not occur within three months, a waiver of intellectual property rights under the Agreement on Trade-Related Aspects of Intellectual Property Rights should come into force immediately."*

At the height of a pandemic, and despite the pattern of obstruction and obfuscation by powerful guardians of the *status quo*, the Panel presented voluntary licensing and technology as a brave frontier, and in giving three months before a waiver of IP rights under TRIPS could come into force, effectively capitulated to the tender sensitivities of those same guardians. Humanity can do better than this.

2.5. Incentives Matter: Overhaul the International Health Regulations

The IHR are "an instrument of international law that is legally-binding on 196 countries, including the 194 WHO Member States."[95] A key element of the IHR is its cautionary stance against the curtailment of international traffic.[96] While the intention is reasonable in principle, it has proven to be astonishingly naïve and impractical in the realities of COVID-19, and it did nothing to prevent or mitigate the chaotic approach to travel restrictions across countries following the outbreak of COVID-19.

The IHR's deficiencies go beyond the example noted above. The WHO should convene purposeful forums to update the IHR, taking into account not only the WHO's traditional comfort zone of normative and lofty statements but a suite of incentives that might be more successful in fostering cooperation among countries, including timely and accurate reporting of disease outbreaks. The incentives to report outbreaks of infectious disease, while favoring the possibility of assistance to control such outbreaks, are at odds with the short-term economic interests of countries that fear restrictions on travel and commerce. Laxminarayan and colleagues note that countries may respond to changing incentives to report outbreaks when possible, and such incentives are probably more important in the long term than assistance for surveillance to ensure prompt reporting of outbreaks.[97]

2.6. Invest in Country and Regional Institutions and Networks

The most striking observations from the first year of the pandemic included the stumbles of the United States Centers for Disease Control and Prevention (US-CDC). The facts initially were not clear, but it is now fair to say that the US-CDC bungled the roll-out of COVID-19 diagnostic tests within the United States.[98] How much of this failure arose from the US-CDC's interaction with the WHO and how much was due to errors within the US-CDC itself remain unclear. Matters reportedly were not helped by the approach of the Trump Administration, which seemed to prioritize political control over enabling the success of the US-CDC, and which seemed unable or unwilling to distinguish science from political spin.

Why this attention to the US-CDC? It is because the US-CDC was widely and highly regarded *as a technical agency* by its partners across the world. Had it not stumbled so badly and become a case study in dysfunction, the US-CDC might have facilitated the work of some other country and national institutes across the world in their responses to COVID-19. Instead, it illustrated the risk to any country or region that would trust a *politically hobbled* US-CDC to be a competent and reliable partner *during acute global crises*.

The strategic lesson for other countries — and regions — is to invest in their own comparable institutions, such as National Public Health Institutes, National Centers for Disease Control and Prevention, and Regional Centers for Disease Control and Prevention. Now that COVID-19 has ravaged the world, the importance of effective institutions for pandemic prevention, rapid detection, and control seems obvious. One such institution is the Africa Centers for Disease Control and Prevention (Africa CDC), which is earning credibility for enabling the continent's response to the COVID-19 pandemic.[99] However, serious commitments to investing in the Africa CDC were not assured in the years that preceded this pandemic. Investing in institutions is not a glamorous undertaking and it takes very serious effort and courage, amidst determined resistance, to secure funding for them. I learned this time and again from first-hand experience.

Even after the devastating Ebola outbreaks in Africa, it was very challenging to secure substantial World Bank financing for the new Africa CDC. The reasons included a failure by otherwise sensible people to grasp the fundamental threats that large and lethal disease outbreaks would pose to lives and economies at the country, regional, and global levels; entrenched aversion to risks of investing in an African regional institution; Kafkaesque processes; a detachment from the changing socio-political narratives and operational realities at the country and regional levels; and a leadership attachment to the Pandemic Emergency Facility (PEF),[100] which subsequently failed despite its razzmatazz. Predicting rain is one thing. The wisdom and fortitude to build a hurricane-resistant ark, instead of merely buying a glitzy but flimsy umbrella, are different matters. It makes strategic and public health sense to invest in mission-critical entities like the Africa CDC. By contrast, it would be wrong to invest additional public money in the failed PEF.[101]

The yellow — if not red — lights were flashing and clear to anyone who paid attention to a dangerous mix of disease outbreak risks — especially but not limited to pathogens crossing from animals to humans, large numbers of people living in mega-cities or traveling across the world, and weaknesses in disease surveillance, detection, and response capacities. With those flashing lights and the institutional lethargy in mind, I relentlessly urged and nudged many colleagues considering the Africa CDC investment program to imagine a massive disease outbreak with far-reaching human and economic damage — and to support an institution that could avert such a disaster through prevention and effective responses. That was one part of a multi-pronged effort to secure funding for the Africa CDC. The merit of the case for investing in the Africa CDC was obvious. If African leaders could claim that they sought support from the World Bank but the World Bank either declined without strong reason or was sluggish in responding to their request, that scenario could damage the World Bank's credibility in an era of emphasis on growing and *protecting* human capital. Several highly professional and courageous colleagues rose to the occasion. I persisted in championing the proposition, the effort continued on multiple and converging fronts, and the World Bank eventually approved funding for the Africa CDC.[102] Upon getting word of the formal approval at 6:15 pm on December 10, 2019, so deep was my relief that I said, "*Nunc dimittis servum tuum, Domine.*"[e]

Although still new and imperfect, the Africa CDC is making a positive difference in the extremely challenging context of COVID-19. There is a more fundamental tide of proactivity rising in Africa. Under the aegis of the African Union, and with the technical leadership and convening power of the Africa CDC, the continent is taking matters into its own hands along multiple dimensions, including The Africa Medical Supplies Platform

---

[e]Now, let your servant go in peace, Lord.

(AMSP),[103] the Africa Regulatory Task Force,[104] and the African Vaccines Acquisition Trust.

The Africa CDC has the capital of sociopolitical legitimacy, which no entity originating outside the continent can muster. Investors with genuine interests in effective disease surveillance and outbreak response functions should encourage and support the Africa CDC so that it develops into a strong, efficient, and effective network in the medium and long terms. Such investments would specifically help to continuously improve its capabilities along multiple dimensions — strategic, technical, administrative, institutional, and financial management. Doing so would help Africa, and given the positive externalities of effective disease prevention and control, it is in the collective self-interest of all continents. It is an example for other regions to consider.

Models of economic growth come with an assumption of *ceteris paribus*. COVID-19 has shown the folly of assuming away the realities of the operating theater. Therefore, investors outside and within Africa, including development finance institutions, would be well advised to get over any bureaucratic lethargy or misinformed squeamishness about investing in such institutions. Those institutions need support precisely because they would perform better if they were strengthened. It is unwise to defer investing in them until they become perfect.

The leadership of the African Union Commission has a big responsibility in this regard. It should transparently ensure operational autonomy for the Africa CDC and avoid self-destructive bureaucratic wars that might suffocate the Africa CDC. These imperatives are not unique to the Africa CDC,[105] but they are especially important for a continent that has just seen the perils of depending on others in matters of health security.

2.7. Governments and Strategic Investments in Industrial Production

In the pre-COVID era, countries of the Global South generally purchased most of their specialized (and in some cases basic) medical equipment and supplies from manufactures in the Global North. The massive spike in demand for diagnostics and ventilators in the first half of 2020, together with the inadequacy of supplies and the breakdowns in logistics and supply chains, highlighted the existential risks inherent in the pre-COVID-19 patterns of trade and dependency. Those existential risks have been amplified by the hoarding of vaccines by the Global North. Within that broad picture, the exposure of Africa's dependence on imported vaccines has been especially glaring.[106]

For countries of the Global South, the solution lies in five concurrent changes.

- First is breaking free from the long-standing orthodox narrative, which holds that governments should not engage in matters such as industrial production, since the market — via private sector businesses — is best placed to do such things. That narrative is incomplete at best, given that governments of the Global North invest extensively in research upon which private businesses often free-ride when they manufacture innovative products.[107,108] The narrative is also misleading because countries of the Global North often subsidize production in areas considered strategic to their interests. Those areas include the aerospace industries and agriculture. For governments of countries in the Global South, there should be no greater strategic interest than the lives of their people. The time is ripe for industrial policy that is at least public health sensitive, and preferably public health focused.[109]
- Second is investing public funds in combinations of subregional and country-based research, development, and manufacturing to meet projected demand in case of future pandemics. The pragmatic question is: *if another massive outbreak occurs in the year 2030, how much of the needs of the Global South should the countries be able to buy at reasonable notice from manufacturing plants located in the Global South?* Even within the Global South, what threshold of concentration of production in any single country or subregion could expose buyer countries to the kind of problem that arose when vaccine exports from India declined in 2021? How the investments are managed is a matter for analysis, vetting, and transparency in the public domain. The ventures could be through different combinations of

public funding and private funding, as could the management and execution of such ventures.

- Third is a modified version of a proposal, by Zerhouni and colleagues, for a system of incentives linked to milestones for innovation and product development.[110] To that system should be added an essential modification: an *ex-ante*, legally binding waiver of all IP rights in the event of major disease outbreaks whose control would benefit from technologies in the agreement.
- Fourth is strengthening supply chains within and across the continents of Africa, Asia, and South America. This includes creating strategic redundancies to be activated in cases of major increases in the demand for medical equipment and supplies.
- Fifth is investing in basic science education at the undergraduate and graduate levels. Countries of the Global South ought to offer tuition-free education to qualified students who major in mathematics, life sciences, engineering, information technology, and medicine. Doing so is an investment in the next generation of home-grown leaders who would capably lead preparations for — and responses to — catastrophic events like COVID-19.

These initiatives are necessary if the Global South is to leave behind its perennial dependency on the Global North for the supply of knowledge- and technology-intensive products. Without these actions, the Global South would self-condemn to being perpetual hewers of wood and drawers of water in the arena of global health.

References

[1] World Health Organization. 2020. WHO Director-General's statement on IHR Emergency Committee on Novel Coronavirus (2019-nCoV). WHO. https://www.who.int/director-general/speeches/detail/who-director-general-s-statement-on-ihr-emergency-committee-on-novel-coronavirus-(2019-ncov). Accessed on March 29, 2021.

[2] World Health Organization. 2021. WHO Coronavirus (COVID-19) Dashboard. https://covid19.who.int. Accessed on July 29, 2021.

[3] Wright L. 2020. *The Plague Year*. New Yorker. https://www.newyorker.com/magazine/2021/01/04/the-plague-year. Accessed on March 29, 2021.

[4] Scott D, Lopez G, Belluz J, Kirby J, Matthews D. *The Pandemic Playbook*. Vox. https://www.vox.com/22381700/pandemic-playbook. Accessed on April 30, 2021.

[5] Global Health Security Index. https://www.ghsindex.org. Accessed on May 10, 2021.

[6] Jamison DT, Lau LJ, Wu KB, *et al.* 2020. Country performance against COVID-19: rankings for 35 countries. *BMJ Global Health*, 5: e003047. https://gh.bmj.com/content/5/12/e003047. Accessed on May 10, 2021.

[7] Horton R. 2020. Why President Trump is wrong about WHO. *The Lancet*, 395(10233), P1330. https://www.thelancet.com/journals/lancet/article/PIIS0140-6736(20)30969-7/fulltext. Accessed on March 29, 2021.

[8] McKee M. 2021. How can we hold political leaders accountable for failures in pandemics? *The BMJ*. 2021. https://blogs.bmj.com/bmj/2021/02/12/martin-mckee-how-can-we-hold-political-leaders-accountable-for-failures-in-pandemics/. Accessed on March 29, 2021.

[9] Frieden T. 2021. On the "mind boggling" interference of the Trump administration during covid-19. *The BMJ*. https://www.bmj.com/content/372/bmj.n565. Accessed on March 29, 2021.

[10] Sparrow A. 2020. Starmer accuses Johnson of 'catastrophic failure of leadership' over England lockdown — as it happened. https://www.theguardian.com/politics/live/2020/nov/02/uk-coronavirus-live-johnson-plays-down-prospect-of-covid-lockdown-extension-ahead-of-facing-tory-critics. Accessed on March 28, 2021.

[11] Londono E, Casado L. 2021. A collapse foretold: How Brazil's Covid-19 outbreak overwhelmed hospitals. https://www.nytimes.com/2021/03/27/world/americas/virus-brazil-bolsonaro.html. Accessed on March 28, 2021.

[12] Taylor L. 2021. 'We are being ignored': Brazil's researchers blame anti-science government for devastating COVID surge. *Nature*. https://www.nature.com/articles/d41586-021-01031-w?utm_source=twt_nnc&utm_medium=social&utm_campaign=naturenews. Accessed on April 29, 2021.

[13] Nicolelis M. 2021. Brazil's pandemic is a 'biological Fukushima' that threatens the entire planet. *Scientific American*. https://www.scientificamerican.com/article/brazils-pandemic-is-a-lsquo-biological-fukushima-rsquo-that-threatens-the-entire-planet/. Accessed on May 7, 2021.

[14] Burke J. 2021. Tanzania's Covid-denying president, John Magufuli, dies aged 61. https://www.theguardian.com/world/2021/mar/17/tanzanias-president-john-magufuli-dies-aged-61. Accessed on March 29, 2021.

[15] *The Lancet.* 2020. COVID-19 in India: The dangers of false optimism. *The Lancet.* Editorial. 396(10255): 867. https://www.thelancet.com/journals/lancet/article/PIIS0140-6736(20)32001-8/fulltext. Accessed on April 29, 2021.

[16] Laxminarayan R. 2021. India's cascading COVID-19 failures. The staggering cost of an unscientific response to the pandemic. *Foreign Affairs.* https://www.foreignaffairs.com/articles/2021-05-26/indias-cascading-covid-19-failures. Accessed on May 26, 2021.

[17] Laxminarayan R. 2021. India's second Covid wave is completely out of control. Opinion. *New York Times.* April 20, 2021. https://www.nytimes.com/2021/04/20/opinion/india-covid-crisis.html. Accessed on April 29, 2021.

[18] Roy A. 2021. We are witnessing a crime against humanity. *The Guardian.* https://www.theguardian.com/news/2021/apr/28/crime-against-humanity-arundhati-roy-india-covid-catastrophe? Accessed on April 29, 2021.

[19] Abbasi K. 2021. India's crisis is everyone's crisis. *BMJ*, 373: n1152. https://www.bmj.com/content/373/bmj.n1152. Accessed on May 6, 2021.

[20] Martin B. 2021. Supply chains and national security. Rand Corporation. https://www.rand.org/blog/2021/04/supply-chains-and-national-security.html. Accessed on April 30, 2021.

[21] The National Academies of Sciences, Engineering, and Medicine. 2021. The security of America's medical product supply chain. Considerations for critical drugs and devices. *Proceedings of a Workshop — In Brief.* April 2021. https://www.nap.edu/catalog/26137/the-security-of-americas-medical-product-supply-chain-considerations-for. Accessed on April 29, 2021.

[22] Colizza V, Barrat A, Barthelemy M, Valleron A, Vespignani A. 2007. Modeling the worldwide spread of pandemic influenza: baseline case and containment interventions. PLoS Medicine, 4(1): e13. https://www.ncbi.nlm.nih.gov/pmc/articles/PMC1779816/. Accessed on April 30, 2021.

[23] Helbing D, Brockman D, Chadefaux T, Donnay K, Blanke U *et al.* 2015. Saving human lives: what complexity science and information systems can contribute. Journal of Statistical Physics, 158(3): 735–781. https://www.ncbi.nlm.nih.gov/pmc/articles/PMC4457089/. Accessed on April 30, 2021.

[24] Hardin G. 1968. The tragedy of the commons. *Science*, 162(3859): 1243–1248. https://science.sciencemag.org/content/162/3859/1243.full. Accessed on March 29, 2021.

[25] What is the ACT-Accelerator. https://www.who.int/initiatives/act-accelerator/about. Accessed on March 28, 2021.

[26] World Health Organization. COVAX. https://www.who.int/initiatives/act-accelerator/covax. Accessed on March 28, 2021.

[27] World Health Organization. 2021. Coronavirus disease (COVID-19): Herd immunity, lockdowns and COVID-19. December 31, 2021. https://www.who.int/news-room/q-a-detail/herd-immunity-lockdowns-and-covid-19. Accessed on April 29, 2021.

[28] Gu Y. Path to herd immunity — COVID-19 vaccine projections. https://covid19-projections.com/path-to-herd-immunity/. Accessed on April 29, 2021.

[29] Cohen J, Kupferschmidt K. 2021. Rich countries cornered COVID-19 vaccine doses. Four strategies to right a 'scandalous inequity'. *Science*. https://www.sciencemag.org/news/2021/05/rich-countries-cornered-covid-19-vaccine-doses-four-strategies-right-scandalous. Accessed on May 27, 2021.

[30] Houston R, Murthy S. 2021. Canada is no global health leader on COVID-19 vaccine equity. *The Lancet*, 397(10287): 1803. https://doi.org/10.1016/S0140-6736(21)00888-6. Accessed on May 14, 2021.

[31] Safi M, Cecco L. 2021. Canada takes Covid vaccines from Covax program despite side deals. https://www.theguardian.com/global-development/2021/feb/03/canada-to-receive-significant-haul-of-covid-vaccines. Accessed on May 24, 2021.

[32] McAdams D, McDade K, Ogbuoji O, Johnson M, Dixit S, Yamey G. 2020. Incentivising wealthy nations to participate in the COVID-19 Vaccine Global Access Facility (COVAX): A game theory perspective. *BMJ Global Health*. https://gh.bmj.com/content/bmjgh/5/11/e003627.full.pdf. Accessed on May 8, 2021.

[33] Cotnam H. 2020. Canada snapping up COVID-19 vaccines at expense of poorer countries, experts say. https://www.cbc.ca/news/canada/ottawa/covid-19-vaccines-canada-covax-insufficient-contribution-global-health-experts-1.5741693. Accessed on March 28, 2021.

[34] Weiland N, Robbins R. 2021. The U.S. is sitting on tens of millions of vaccine doses the world needs. https://www.nytimes.com/2021/03/11/us/politics/coronavirus-astrazeneca-united-states.html? Accessed on March 28, 2021.

[35] Emanuel E, Fabre C, Halliday D, Leland R, Buchanan A, Tan K, Chan SY. 2021. How many vaccine doses can nations ethically hoard? The case for sharing supplies prior to reaching herd immunity. https://www.foreignaffairs.com/articles/world/2021-03-09/how-many-vaccine-doses-can-nations-ethically-hoard. Accessed on March 29, 2021.

[36] Boffey D. 2021. 'Lack of perspective': Why Ursula von der Leyen's EU vaccine strategy is failing. *The Guardian*. https://www.theguardian.com/world/2021/mar/28/jean-claude-juncker-and-dominic-cummings-unite-on-ursula-von-der-leyen-eu-stupid-vaccine-war. Accessed on March 28, 2021.

[37] *Financial Times*. 'Everyone's scrambling and hoarding': Europe's vaccine blunders.   https://www.ft.com/content/53629923-47c9-4047-8022-031010d39e18. Accessed on March 28, 2021.

[38] Sevastopulo D, Kazmin A. 2021. US and Asia allies plan Covid vaccine strategy to counter China. *Financial Times*. https://www.ft.com/content/1dc04520-c2fb-4859-9821-c405f51f8586. Accessed on March 29, 2021.

[39] Henley J. 2021. Is Russia's Covid vaccine anything more than a political weapon? *The Guardian*. https://www.theguardian.com/society/2021/apr/30/is-russias-covid-vaccine-anything-more-than-a-political-weapon-sputnik-v. Accessed on April 30, 2021.

[40] Mazzucato M. 2021. Capitalism won't save us from Covid, no matter what Boris Johnson might think. *The Guardian*. https://www.theguardian.com/commentisfree/2021/mar/27/capitalism-covid-boris-johnson-uk-vaccine-state-funding. Accessed on March 28, 2021.

[41] Tharoor K. 2021. The vaccine rollout makes it clear: The randomness of nationality still determines our lives. https://www.theguardian.com/commentisfree/2021/mar/02/vaccine-rollout-nationality-covid-jab-poorer-countries? Accessed on March 28, 2021.

[42] Bump JB, Baum F, Sakornsin M, Yates R, Hofman K. 2021. Political economy of covid-19: extractive, regressive, competitive. *The BMJ*, 372. doi: https://doi.org/10.1136/bmj.n73. Accessed on January 29, 2021.

[43] Phillips T, Giuffrida A. 2020. 'Doctor diplomacy': Cuba seeks to make its mark in Europe amid Covid-19 crisis. *The Guardian*. https://www.theguardian.com/world/2020/may/06/doctor-diplomacy-cuba-seeks-to-make-its-mark-in-europe-amid-covid-19-crisis. Accessed on April 29, 2021.

[44] International Monetary Fund. Fiscal Monitor Update. January 2021. https://www.imf.org/en/Publications/FM/Issues/2021/01/20/fiscal-monitor-update-january-2021. Accessed on March 28, 2021.

[45] Gopinath G. 2021. Drawing Further Apart: Widening Gaps in the Global Recovery. International Monetary Fund. https://blogs.imf.org/2021/07/27/drawing-further-apart-widening-gaps-in-the-global-recovery/. Accessed on July 28, 2021.

[46] Usher A. 2020. South Africa and India push for COVID-19 patents ban. *The Lancet*. https://www.thelancet.com/journals/lancet/article/PIIS0140-6736(20)32581-2/fulltext. Accessed on March 28, 2021.

[47] Irwin A. 2021. What it will take to vaccinate the world against COVID-19. *Nature*. https://www.nature.com/articles/d41586-021-00727-3. Accessed on March 28, 2021.

[48] Kuchler H. 2021. Covid vaccines spur global fight over intellectual property. *Financial Times.* https://www.ft.com/content/b0f42409-6fdf-43eb-96c7-d166e090ab99. Accessed on May 4, 2021.

[49] Ubl S, Ricks D. 2021. Untitled. Letter to President Joseph Biden. March 5, 2021. PhRMA. Washington, DC. https://phrma.org/-/media/Project/PhRMA/PhRMA-Org/PhRMA-Org/PDF/P-R/20210305-PhRMA-Letter-to-President-Biden.pdf?utm_source=STAT+Newsletters&utm_campaign=f752eeaf52-EMAIL_CAMPAIGN_2021_03_08_10_19&utm_medium=email&utm_term=0_8cab1d7961-f752eeaf52-152708089. Accessed on April 29, 2021.

[50] Thambietty S, McMahon A, McDonagh L, Kang HY, Dutfield G. 2021. The TRIPS intellectual property waiver proposal: Creating the right incentives in patent law and politics to end the COVID-19 pandemic. LSE Legal Studies Working Paper (forthcoming, 2021). https://papers.ssrn.com/sol3/papers.cfm?abstract_id=3851737&download=yes. Accessed on May 26, 2021.

[51] Mazzucato M, Ghosh J, Torreele E. 2021. Intellectual property and COVID-19. *The Economist.* April 20, 2021. https://www.economist.com/by-invitation/2021/04/20/mariana-mazzucato-jayati-ghosh-and-els-torreele-on-waiving-covid-patents. Accessed on April 29, 2021.

[52] Yadav P, Weintraub R. 2021. 4 strategies to boost the global supply of Covid-19 vaccines. *Harvard Business Review.* https://hbr.org/2021/05/4-strategies-to-boost-the-global-supply-of-covid-19-vaccines. Accessed on May 6, 2021.

[53] Jha P, Jamison DT, Watkins DA, Bell J. 2021. A global compact to counter vaccine nationalism. *The Lancet.* https://doi.org/10.1016/S0140-6736(21)01105-3. Accessed on May 18, 2021.

[54] Lawder D. 2021. Vaccine IP waiver could take months for WTO to negotiate-experts. *Reuters.* https://www.reuters.com/world/china/vaccine-ip-waiver-could-take-months-wto-negotiate-experts-2021-05-06/ Accessed on May 6, 2021.

[55] Sengupta S. 2021. U.S. is under pressure to release vaccine supplies as India faces deadly surge. https://www.nytimes.com/2021/04/24/climate/inda-covid-vaccines.html. Accessed on April 29, 2021.

[56] Rogers K, Stolberg S. 2021. U.S. to send virus-ravaged India materials for vaccines. https://www.nytimes.com/2021/04/25/us/politics/india-us-coronavirus.html. Accessed on April 29, 2021.

[57] Office of The United States Trade Representative. 2021. Statement from Ambassador Katherine Tai on the Covid-19 trips waiver. https://ustr.gov/about-us/policy-offices/press-office/press-releases/2021/may/statement-ambassador-katherine-tai-covid-19-trips-waiver. Accessed on May 5, 2021.

[58] IFPMA. 2021. IFPMA statement on WTO TRIPS intellectual property waiver. https://www.ifpma.org/resource-centre/ifpma-statement-on-wto-trips-intellectual-property-waiver/. Accessed on May 6, 2021.

[59] Stevis-Gridness M. 2021. E.U. leader says bloc is willing to discuss patent waiver for Covid vaccines. *New York Times*. https://www.nytimes.com/2021/05/06/world/europe/coronavirus-vaccine-patent-eu.html. Accessed on May 6, 2021.

[60] Borger J. 2021. US-Germany Rift as Berlin opposes plan to ditch Covid vaccine patents. *The Guardian*. https://www.theguardian.com/world/2021/may/06/us-germany-rift-covid-vaccine-patent-waivers. Accessed on May 6, 2021.

[61] *BBC*. 2021. Covid: US backs waiver on vaccine patents to boost supply. https://www.bbc.com/news/world-us-canada-57004302. Accessed on May 6, 2021.

[62] *BBC*. 2021. Covid: Germany rejects US-backed proposal to waive vaccine patents. https://www.bbc.com/news/world-europe-57013096. Accessed on May 6, 2021.

[63] Boffey D, Connolly K. 2021. Macron voices concerns over COVID vaccines patent waiver. *The Guardian*. https://www.theguardian.com/world/2021/may/07/macron-voices-concerns-over-covid-vaccines-patent-waiver. Accessed on May 6, 2021.

[64] Landler M, Castle S. 2021. U.K. and France call in the navy, sort of, in channel islands fishing dispute. *New York Times*. https://www.nytimes.com/2021/05/06/world/europe/uk-france-jersey-fishing.html. Accessed on May 6, 2021.

[65] Obregon L. 2018. Empire, racial capitalism and international law: The case of manumitted Haiti and the recognition debt. *Leiden Journal of International Law*, 31(3): 597–615. https://doi.org/10.1017/S0922156518000225. Accessed on May 10, 2021.

[66] Maxmen A. 2021. Why some researchers oppose unrestricted sharing of coronavirus genome data. *Nature*. https://www.nature.com/articles/d41586-021-01194-6. Accessed on May 10, 2021.

[67] Pakenham T. *The Scramble for Africa. The White Man's Conquest of the Dark Continent from 1876 to 1912*. 1991. New York: Random House. pp. 239–256.

[68] Montreal Holocaust Museum. Herero genocide in Namibia. https://museeholocauste.ca/en/resources-training/herero-genocide-namibia/. Accessed on May 26, 2021.

[69] United States Department of State. The Berlin airlift, 1948–1949. https://history.state.gov/milestones/1945-1952/berlin-airlift. Accessed on May 6, 2021.

[70] Putnam T. 2013. The real meaning of *Ich Bin ein Berliner. The Atlantic*. https://www.theatlantic.com/magazine/archive/2013/08/the-real-meaning-of-ich-bin-ein-berliner/309500/. Accessed on May 17, 2021.

[71] Gostin LO. 2021. Health injustice: The dominant global narrative of our time. *Global Health Governance*, XI(1) (Special Symposium Issue 2021) http://www.ghgj.org. https://blogs.shu.edu/ghg/files/2021/05/Spring-2021-Issue.pdf. Accessed on May 17, 2021.

[72] Kickbusch I, Franz C, Holzscheiter A, Hunger I, Jahn A *et al.* 2017. Germany's expanding role in global health. *The Lancet*, 390(10097): P898–912. https://www.thelancet.com/journals/lancet/article/PIIS0140-6736(17)31460-5/fulltext. Accessed on May 6, 2021.

[73] Horton R. 2021. Offline: What is the UK for? *The Lancet*, 397(1027): P654. https://www.thelancet.com/journals/lancet/article/PIIS0140-6736(21)00431-1/fulltext. Accessed on May 6, 2021.

[74] Persad G, Lynch HF. 2021. Millions of vaccines are about to expire. The U.S. might just let them go to waste. *Washington Post*. https://www.washingtonpost.com/outlook/2021/07/27/coronavirus-vaccine-waste/. Accessed on July 28, 2021.

[75] Fallah M. 2021. Remember Ebola: stop mass COVID deaths in Africa. *Nature*. https://www.nature.com/articles/d41586-021-01964-2. Accessed on July 28, 2021.

[76] Doherty B, Hurst D, Lyons K. 2021. Coercion or altruism: Is China using its Covid vaccines to wield global power? *The Guardian*. https://www.theguardian.com/australia-news/2021/mar/28/coercion-or-altruism-is-china-using-its-covid-vaccines-to-wield-global-power. Accessed on May 13, 2021.

[77] Huang Y. Vaccine diplomacy is paying off for China. *Foreign Affairs*. https://www.foreignaffairs.com/articles/china/2021-03-11/vaccine-diplomacy-paying-china. Accessed on May 13, 2021.

[78] Gates RM. 2020. *Exercise of Power*. Alfred A. Knopf. p. 365.

[79] Pyle R. 1990. Mandela explains support for PLO, Gadhafi, Castro with PM-Mandela, Bjt. *AP News*. https://apnews.com/article/f7cc35e2e78be9a2b-d132ebdedc0aaeb. Accessed on May 12, 2021.

[80] Editorial Board of the Washington Post. 2021. A patent-free 'people's vaccine' is not the best way to help poor countries. *Washington Post*. https://www.washingtonpost.com/opinions/global-opinions/how-to-help-the-poorest-countries-get-vaccinated/2021/05/03/18d5b79a-ac3a-11eb-acd3-24b44a57093a_story.html. Accessed on May 4, 2021.

[81] Allen A. 2020. For billion-dollar COVID vaccines, basic government-funded science laid the groundwork. *Scientific American*. https://www.scientificamerican.com/article/for-billion-dollar-covid-vaccines-basic-government-funded-science-laid-the-groundwork/. Accessed on May 5, 2021.

[82] Meade J, Li S. Fall 2015. Strategic corporate tax lobbying. *JATA American Accounting Association*, 37(2): 23–48. https://www.bauer.uh.edu/jmeade/articles/JATA%20Fall_2015.pdf. Accessed on May 5, 2021.

[83] Wamsley L. 2021. FDA inspection finds numerous problems at facility intended to make J&J vaccine. *National Public Radio.* https://www.npr.org/sections/coronavirus-live-updates/2021/04/21/989549809/fda-inspection-finds-numerous-problems-at-facility-intended-to-make-j-j-vaccine. Accessed on May 6, 2021.

[84] Department of Health and Human Services. Food and Drug Administration. 2021. Observations made by the FDA Representative during inspection of Emergent Manufacturing Operations Baltimore LLC. https://www.fda.gov/media/147762/download?utm_medium=email&utm_source=govdelivery. Accessed on May 24, 2021.

[85] The White House. 2021. Fact Sheet: The American jobs plan. https://www.whitehouse.gov/briefing-room/statements-releases/2021/03/31/fact-sheet-the-american-jobs-plan/. Accessed on May 5, 2021.

[86] Gelinas N. 2007. Lessons of Boston's big dig. America's most ambitious infrastructure project inspired engineering marvels — and colossal mismanagement. *City Journal.* https://www.city-journal.org/html/lessons-boston's-big-dig-13049.html. Accessed on May 4, 2021.

[87] Africa Centers for Disease Control and Prevention. 2021. Virtual conference: Expanding Africa's vaccine manufacturing — Africa CDC. https://africacdc.org/event/virtual-conference-expanding-africas-vaccine-manufacturing/. Accessed on May 4, 2021.

[88] Agyarko R. 2021. A new era of vaccine sovereignty in Africa beckons. *The Mail and Guardian.* https://mg.co.za/africa/2021-04-14-a-new-era-of-vaccine-sovereignty-in-africa-beckons/. Accessed on May 4, 2021.

[89] Editorial Board of *The Washington Post.* 2021. It's time to apply warp speed to vaccinate the globe. May 8, 2021. https://www.washingtonpost.com/opinions/global-opinions/its-time-to-apply-warp-speed-to-vaccinate-the-globe/2021/05/07/2e57c2c4-af60-11eb-acd3-24b44a57093a_story.html. Accessed on May 11, 2021.

[90] European Commission. 2021. Statement by President von der Leyen following the Global Health Summit. https://ec.europa.eu/commission/presscorner/detail/en/statement_21_2622. Accessed on May 26, 2021.

[91] Nature. 2021. A patent waiver on COVID vaccines is right and fair. Editorial. *Nature.* https://www.nature.com/articles/d41586-021-01242-1. Accessed on May 26, 2021.

[92] Lawder D. 2021. World Bank opposes vaccine intellectual property waiver as WTO talks resume. Reuters. https://www.reuters.com/business/healthcarepharmaceuticals/world-bank-chief-says-does-not-support-vaccine-intellectualproperty-waiver-wto-2021-06-08/. Accessed on June 9, 2021.

[93] Fidler D. January 2008. Influenza virus samples, international law, and global health diplomacy. *Emerging Infectious Diseases*, 14(1). https://wwwnc.cdc.gov/eid/article/14/1/07-0700_article. Accessed on March 28, 2021.

[94] The Independent Panel for Pandemic Preparedness and Response. 2021. COVID-19: Make it the last pandemic. https://theindependentpanel.org/wp-content/uploads/2021/05/COVID-19-Make-it-the-Last-Pandemic_final.pdf. Accessed on May 13, 2021.

[95] World Health Organization. International health regulations. https://www.who.int/health-topics/international-health-regulations#tab=tab_1. Accessed on March 28, 2021.

[96] Habibi R, Burci G, de Campos T, Chirwa D *et al.* 2020. Do not violate the International Health Regulations during the COVID-19 outbreak. *The Lancet*, 395(10225). https://doi.org/10.1016/S0140-6736(20)30373-1. Accessed on March 28, 2021.

[97] Laxminarayan R, Reif J, Malani A. 2014. Incentives for reporting disease outbreaks. *PLoS One*, 9(3): e90290. https://pubmed.ncbi.nlm.nih.gov/24603414/. Accessed on March 29, 2021.

[98] Guillen D. 2021. U.S. exceptionalism created deadly COVID-19 failures. *Foreign Policy*. https://foreignpolicy.com/2021/03/18/us-exceptionalism-covid-19-deaths/. Accessed on March 28, 2021.

[99] Resolve to save lives. COVID-19 in Africa. Case study. https://preventepidemics.org/epidemics-that-didnt-happen/covid-19-africa/. Accessed on May 31, 2021.

[100] Alloway T, Vossos T. 2020. How pandemic bonds became the world's most controversial investment. *Bloomberg*. https://www.bloomberg.com/news/features/2020-12-09/covid-19-finance-how-the-world-bank-s-pandemic-bonds-became-controversial. Accessed on May 31, 2021.

[101] Ritchie E, Plant M. 2020. A good idea executed badly: Why the World Bank should not renew the pandemic emergency facility insurance window. https://www.cgdev.org/blog/good-idea-executed-badly-why-world-bank-should-not-renew-pandemic-emergency-facility-insurance. Accessed on May 16, 2021.

[102] The World Bank. *Africa Union, Ethiopia and Zambia — Africa Centers for Disease Control and Prevention Regional Investment Financing Project* (English). Washington, DC: World Bank Group. https://documents1.worldbank.org/curated/en/550521576292519493/pdf/Africa-Union-Ethiopia-and-Zambia-Africa-Centres-for-Disease-Control-and-Prevention-Regional-Investment-Financing-Project.pdf. Accessed on May 31, 2021.

[103] Africa Medical Supplies Platform. https://amsp.africa/about-us/. Accessed on March 29, 2021.

[104] Africa CDC. 2021. https://africacdc.org/download/african-union-and-the-africa-centers-for-disease-control-and-preventions-africa-regulatory-taskforce-has-endorsed-the-emergency-used-authorization-for-janssen-covid-19-vaccine/. Accessed on March 28, 2021.

[105] Salwa J, Robertson C. 2021. Designing an independent public health agency. *NEJM.* https://www.nejm.org/doi/full/10.1056/NEJMp2033970. Accessed on May 5, 2021.

[106] *The Economist.* 2021. Covid-19 has exposed Africa's dependence on vaccines from abroad. https://amp.economist.com/weeklyedition/2021-05-08. Accessed on May 8, 2021.

[107] Mazzucato M. 2015. *The Entrepreneurial State: Debunking Public vs. Private Sector Myths.* New York, NY: Hachette Book Group, Inc.

[108] Castillo J, Ajuka A, Athey S, Baker A, Budish E *et al.* 2021. Market design to accelerate covid19 vaccine supply. *Science*, 371(6534): 1107–1109. https://science.sciencemag.org/content/371/6534/1107.full. Accessed on March 28, 2021.

[109] Torreele E, Kazatchkine M, Mariana M. 2021. Preparing for the next pandemic requires public health focused industrial policy. *BMJ.* https://blogs.bmj.com/bmj/2021/04/01/preparing-for-the-next-pandemic-requires-public-health-focused-industrial-policy/. Accessed on April 30, 2021.

[110] Zerhouni W, Nabel GJ, Zerhouni E. 2020. Patents, economics, and pandemics. *Science*, 368(6495). https://science.sciencemag.org/content/368/6495/1035/tab-pdf. Accessed on April 29, 2021.

Chapter 3

Markets, Governments, and Global Health

"The absurd consequences of focusing fanatically on a single idea, like free markets and equality, instead of on measuring performance and doing what works are obvious to anyone who spends time looking at the realities of life in Cuba and the United States."

—Hans Rosling[a]

Synopsis

This chapter is the first of three on the roles of markets, the private sector, and governments in global health. It provides an overview of principles and unresolved issues of relevance to the practice of global health. Discussions about markets and governments often evoke strongly held beliefs and positions, particularly on appropriate roles of the private sector and public policy. The strengths of these beliefs and positions come from varying combinations of theoretical doctrines, empirical evidence, anecdotes, ideologies, and grand myths. These combinations have practical consequences for global health, as they help explain the origins of health systems in different parts of the world and the dynamics of Development Assistance for Health (DAH). It is important to look at — and beyond — the failures of governments and markets,

---

[a]Rosling H. 2018. *Factfulness*. New York: Flatiron Books. pp. 194–195.

with attention to just what it is that decision makers are optimizing for. Doing so paves the way for measured considerations of equity of access to technologies and services, and for careful distinctions between means and ends.

3.1. Beyond Government Failures and Market Failures

Markets and the commercial private sector represent many things, and different things to various constituencies, in the practice of global health. This is especially so for the architecture and practice of DAH. To the extent that markets are seen as means to specified ends, they hold much promise, albeit with caveats. To the extent that markets are seen as ends unto themselves, they present enormous perils. For irredeemably anti-market ideologues, including but not limited to some in the international NGO community, the commercial private sector is a gift that keeps giving: it can be vilified as unspeakably evil and the bashers do not have to propose anything beyond ideology of the omnipotent and omniscient government, evidence to the contrary be damned.

Stiglitz notes that the market is constrained pareto efficient only under highly idealized circumstances,[1] or, in plain speak, "Adam Smith's invisible hand — the idea that free markets lead to efficiency as if guided by unseen forces — is invisible, at least in part, because it is not there."[2] Schefler is more direct:

> "One of the best-kept secrets in economics is that there is no case for the invisible hand. After more than a century trying to prove the opposite, economic theorists investigating the matter finally concluded in the 1970s that there is no reason to believe markets are led, as if by an invisible hand, to an optimal equilibrium — or any equilibrium at all. But the message never got through to their supposedly practical colleagues who so eagerly push advice about almost anything. Most never even heard what the theorists said, or else resolutely ignored it."[3]

Hsiao and Heller laid out key characteristics of practical value to those working in global health.[4] The health sector has major market failures. For example, the supply side dominates the demand side in the health services market, with asymmetry of information between trained service providers and patients. Without any regulatory intervention, health workers can use their monopolistic powers to provide more services than the patient truly needs. They can do so while setting high prices. The consequence is cost inflation with poorer quality of services.

Given these health market failures, is the practical solution for governments to undertake end-to-end control and management of the health care system? The experience of the formerly socialist economies of Eastern Europe and the USSR provides evidence to the contrary.[5] This brings us to the matter of Government Failure, which arises when inappropriate government intervention creates inefficiencies.[6] Global health practice is rife with highly charged positions about what governments must do or must not do. Often lost in the discussions is the question of what type of government actions are most appropriate and feasible in which setting, and why. Blank notes that consumers may care more about quality than they do about price. If quality is readily observable and measurable, the government can, in principle, regulate private providers to assure standards are met. That assumes the government has the real-life capacity to do so. In practice, some government ministries of health in the Global South can neither prepare their own budgets without "technical assistance" nor effectively regulate and supervise public sector providers. Regulating private providers is not feasible in such settings, at least not for the near future.[7]

In "The failure of private health services: COVID-19 induced crises in low- and middle-income country (LMIC) health systems," Williams and colleagues contend that for decades, governments and development partners promoted "neoliberal policies" in the health sector in many LMICs, largely motivated by the belief that governments in these countries were too weak to provide all the health services necessary to meet population needs. But, are the governments demonstrably able to provide all these services? How often is government responsibility for *ensuring the provision* of health services conflated with the *actual provision* of those services? There is nothing inherently governmental in the actual provision of most health services that individuals receive in health centers and hospitals. Nevertheless, Williams and colleagues usefully identified how market failure and failures of redistribution have caused the rise of three crises in those health systems: a financial and liquidity crisis among private providers, a crisis of service provision and pricing, and a crisis in state–provider relations. Their conclusion merits attention because the COVID-19 pandemic has exposed important failures of the public–private models of health systems and provides an opportunity to rethink the future orientation of national health systems and commitments toward UHC.[8] Those conclusions are in sync with some considerations in Chapter 2 of this book.

The angst is not limited to LMICs. Why would Americans tend to rebel when their government tells them what to do, but be rather acquiescent when their employers dictate to them, including potential mandates for COVID-19 vaccines? Setting aside the possible reason that many Americans did not elect their representatives (the representatives chose the voters via gerrymandering), but they chose their employers, is Parmet on to something about the privatization of public health?[9] If so, is that inherently good or bad?

The tension between the profit-maximizing objective of pharmaceutical companies and the public health-maximizing duty of governments has been a recurring theme regarding, among others, HIV/AIDS, Hepatitis C, and now COVID-19. This is often portrayed as a "misalignment between economic incentives driving the industry versus benefit to the public."[10] The question is whether that misalignment is truly inherent or contrived. To the extent that taxpayers fund the basic science research that underpins innovations by many large pharmaceutical companies, the public subsidizes those companies. But companies pocket most or all the profits that accrue from the monopolies conferred by patents, and then argue that patent waivers would stifle innovation!

In a rational framework, the companies should pay royalties to the public that funded the basic research *and* pay corporate taxes on their profits. But the system is warped by lobbying. In the United States, from 1999 to 2018, the pharmaceutical and health product industry recorded US$4.7 billion — an average of US$233 million per year — in lobbying expenditures at the federal level, more than any other industry. In years with referendums on reforms in drug pricing and regulation, there were major increases in contributions to groups that opposed or supported the reforms.[11] Far from being rational, the system is rigged in favor of the companies. Trust cartoonists to get the point; one showed a pharmaceutical industry lobbyist inviting legislators for a tutorial on how laws are made.

An important problem with a framework based on mitigating government and market failures is that it is too self-limiting and ignores a more profound role of government. In *The Entrepreneurial State,* Mazzucato argues that in certain cases the state has been key to creating and shaping markets, not only fixing market failures, and identified four dimensions of thinking big about mission-oriented policies, as follows:[12]

(1) Empowering governments to chart and invest in a direction for change.
(2) Adopting a new approach of evaluating public spending that considers its courage to push markets into new areas, instead of the traditional view that the public and private actors must crowd out each other in existing markets.
(3) Allowing for experimentation, learning, and failure in public organizations.
(4) Identifying how governments and taxpayers can reap some of the rewards (read: profits) from the upside, instead of merely de-risking the downside.

While these four dimensions were defined in terms of innovative technologies, they are relevant to much of the discourse on global health.

3.2. Optimizing for Equity

From the perspective of translating public policy into practice, it is important to identify the priority for which a government seeks to optimize. Most governments have formally committed to achieving UHC,[13] combining coverage of the population with essential health services, ensuring the quality of services delivered, and avoiding financial hardship for those receiving services. Therefore, rational policy makers in this case would be neither ideologues of the free market nor ideologues of government command and control. Instead, they would be most concerned with what combination of government action and market forces would provide the biggest benefit for most people along the road to UHC, given the fiscal constraints. They would not use price as the primary rationing tool, especially in situations where private out-of-pocket expenditures are already high and causing individuals and households to experience financial hardship.

It follows that governments seeking to stretch scarce resources to disproportionately benefit the poorer, more marginalized, and harder-to-reach segments of their population would primarily emphasize equity while secondarily seeking to improve their efficiency. Markets, insofar as the supply side comes from the commercial private sector, are better at the efficiency that drives profit maximization. Therefore, since market competition can address only the efficiency challenge, governments have to be responsible for the equitable financing and distribution of essential health goods.[4]

Among global health practitioners, there is no universally settled, real-life clarity on the roles of government and the private sector where the public policy goal is set to optimize for equity. Regarding affordability, Klein and Hadjimichael note that desired levels of service for the poor could be achieved by targeting subsidies through a variety of approaches to the poor while contracting out provision.[14] Even such targeting would happen in a broader theater with multiple and often competing interest groups. In practice, policy makers have only a few strategic levers to deploy, and their use of those levers is often constrained by political considerations. The levers include setting directions, allocation of scarce resources amidst competing priorities, provision of incentives for better performance, oversight of the public sector and regulation of the private sector, and establishment of mutually beneficial initiatives among countries.

3.3. Access to Health Technologies and Services

The pursuit of effective coverage[15] in UHC is central to achieving equity and related to broader challenges of access. Regarding technologies, Frost and Reich's Access Framework consists of four A's[16]: architecture, availability, affordability, and adoption. They contend that getting the four activity streams right can improve access to health technologies, and that a deeper understanding of the facilitators, barriers, and key actors involved in achieving architecture, availability, affordability, and adoption is necessary for better access planning. The reader is encouraged to keep this in mind when reading the next two chapters.

A key message from this chapter is that provided public policy is clear about its goals, ideological purity is not a virtue in the pursuit of those goals. It is far more prudent to take the empiricist's approach: set hypotheses, experiment, measure, evaluate, learn, and improve in iterative cycles. Prahalad provided examples of business success stories from "the Bottom of the Pyramid."[17] Some of them, Aravind Eye Care, The Jaipur Foot Story, and Health Alerts for All, are in or largely about health services. Once freed of the shackles of reflex rejection of anything governmental or anything market-driven, it becomes possible to engage in productive, evidence-based policy making, policy translation, and program implementation that makes the best use of public sector and private sector capabilities to benefit people at the bottom of the pyramid of wealth and opportunity.

Bennett and colleagues identified three themes from a survey of global stakeholders on their perceptions of the pressure points in health markets that could trigger positive change across the market. They reported the following:[18]

- private for-profit providers were unlikely to serve the poor if left on their own, and the only ways to get such providers to reach this market was through subsidies or through the expansion of health insurance schemes;
- health markets in LMICs continue to be plagued by poor quality, unnecessary care, and nontransparent pricing, with regulatory failures being important aspects of the problem; and
- the evidence base on many health market issues was relatively weak.

3.4. Ends versus Means

So far, so good. But government responsibility for an outcome is different from government suitability for the direct execution of activities leading to that outcome. All too often in global health, interest groups conflate public ends with exclusively public means. This is not exclusive to advocacy groups in the Global South. Some of the most ardent proponents of governmental command-and-control approach to public health goals are prominent NGOs that come from the Global North to work — and ostensibly speak on behalf of *the natives* — in the Global South. It is remarkable that such governmental absolutism is not the status in most countries of Western Europe and North America from whence these NGOs come, and their governments have much higher capacities for public administration than most governments of LICs and MICs. The collapse of the former Soviet Union shows the perils of a government-alone-must-do-everything mentality. Therefore, it is odd that some of those NGOs from the Global North advocate for approaches that require governments of LICs and MICs to directly and comprehensively perform feats of administration and implementation that their home countries cannot and do not directly perform. Such faulty thinking obviates opportunities that might exist to use mixtures of public and private capacities and to prudently use private means to pursue public ends via variations of strategic purchasing,[19] removing any room for the strategic purchasing of supply chain management and clinical service delivery, neither of which is inherently governmental.

3.4.1 Public–Private partnerships

Policy makers often have just a few levers within their purview, with time-bound tenures that could be cut short by any number of factors. Faced with the strengths and failures of both governments and markets, agnostic regarding the specific means, and seeking to optimize for equity, what might policy makers do amidst resource constraints? Many have either turned to or are considering public–private partnerships (PPPs) for solutions. But how promising are they? Does the reality live up to the promise? What determines successes and failures? Above all, what is good enough from a public policy perspective?

The PPP Knowledge Lab provides a succinct overview of key themes and challenges of relevance to health.[20] In principle, PPPs can combine the strengths of the public and private sectors to expand resources available for service delivery, improve management capacity, extend the reach (coverage) and richness (quality) of services to underserved or hard-to-reach populations, spur innovation, and improve transparency. They might even enhance efficiency in ways that help to curb corruption.[21]

The following challenges loom large in designing and running PPPs: clarity on the role of government, government capacity to negotiate and manage contracts, performance measurement, budget predictability, affordability, regulatory certainty, private sector capacity to engage with government, and political sustainability across successive governments.

3.4.2 In practice

What do all these mean in practice? The following two chapters provide detailed explorations of two situations that illustrate the principles, exciting opportunities, gains, and challenges highlighted in this chapter. The reader is encouraged to study them with attention to the convergences and divergences between theory and practice. For current and potential investors in health at the global, regional, or country levels, the questions are:

- what are you optimizing for, and
- what is the appropriate and feasible combination of levers to achieve your goals?

References

[1] Stiglitz JE. 1991. The invisible hand and modern welfare economics. NBER Working Paper Number 3641. https://www.nber.org/papers/w3641. Accessed on January 16, 2021.

[2] Stiglitz J. 2002. There is no invisible hand. https://www.theguardian.com/education/2002/dec/20/highereducation.uk1. Accessed on January 16, 2021.

[3] Schefler J. 2012. There is no invisible hand. *Harvard Business Review*. https://hbr.org/2012/04/there-is-no-invisible-hand. Accessed on January 16, 2021.

[4] Hsiao WC, Heller PS. 2007. *What Macroeconomists Should Know about Health Care Policy*. International Monetary Fund. http://dx.doi.org/10.5089/9781589066182.058. Accessed on January 16, 2021.

[5] Preker AS, Adeyi OO. 2005. Health care. In Barr N (Editor). *Labor Markets and Social Policy in Central and Eastern Europe. The Accession and Beyond*. Washington, DC: The World Bank. p. 171–187.

[6] Winston C. 2006. Government failure vs. market failure: microeconomics policy research and government performance. https://www.brookings.edu/research/government-failure-vs-market-failure-microeconomics-policy-research-and-government-performance/. Accessed on January 16, 2021.

[7] Blank R M. March 2000. When can public policy makers rely on private markets? The effective provision of social services. *The Economic Journal*, 110(462): C34–C49. https://academic.oup.com/ej/article-abstract/110/462/C34/5140010. Accessed on January 301, 2021.

[8] Williams OD, Yung KC, Grepin K. 2021. The failure of private health services: COVID-19 induced crises in low- and middle-income country (LMIC) health systems. *Global Public Health*. https://www.tandfonline.com/doi/full/10.1080/17441692.2021.1874470. Accessed on January 30, 2021.

[9] Parmet W. 2021. Employers' vaccine mandates are representative of America's failed approach to public health. *We can't rely on the private sector to protect the common good.* The Atlantic. https://www.theatlantic.com/ideas/archive/2021/02/privatization-public-health/617918/. Accessed on March 24, 2021.

[10] Zerhouni W, Nabel GJ, Zerhouni E. June 5, 2020. Patents, economics, and pandemics. *Science*, 368(6495). https://science.sciencemag.org/content/368/6495/1035/tab-pdf. Accessed on April 29, 2021.

[11] Wouters O. May, 2020. Lobbying expenditures and campaign contributions by the pharmaceutical and health product industry in the United States, 1999–2018. *JAMA Internal Medicine*, 180(5): 1–10. https://www.ncbi.nlm.nih.gov/pmc/articles/PMC7054854/. Accessed on April 30, 2021.

[12] Mazzucato M. 2015. *The Entrepreneurial State: Debunking Public vs. Private Sector Myths.* New York, NY: Hachette Book Group, Inc.

[13] United Nations General Assembly. Political declaration of the high-level meeting on universal health coverage. *Resolution adopted by the General Assembly on October 10, 2019.* p. 1. https://undocs.org/en/A/RES/74/2. Accessed on December 18, 2019.

[14] Klein MU, Hadjimichael B. 2003. *The Private Sector in Development: Entrepreneurship, Regulation, and Competitive Disciplines.* The International Bank for Reconstruction and Development. pp. 87–125.

[15] GBD 2019 Universal Health Coverage Collaborators. 2020. Measuring universal health coverage based on an index of effective coverage of health services in 204 countries and territories, 1990–2019: a systematic analysis for the Global Burden of Disease Study 2019. *Lancet*, 396: 1250–1284. Published Online August 27, 2020. https://www.thelancet.com/journals/lancet/article/PIIS0140-6736(20)30750-9/fulltext. Accessed January 30, 2021.

[16] Frost LJ, Reich MR. 2008. *Access: How Do Good Health Technologies Get to Poor People in Poor Countries?* Cambridge, MA: Harvard Center for Population and Development Studies. pp. 15–38.

[17] Prahalad CK. 2006. *The Fortune at the Bottom of the Pyramid.* Upper Saddle River: Wharton School Publishing.

[18] Bennett S, Bloom G, Knezovich J, Peters DH. 2014. The future of health markets. *Globalization and Health,* 10(51). https://link.springer.com/article/10.1186/1744-8603-10-51. Accessed on January 30, 2021.

[19] Preker AS, Langenbrunner JC, Belli PC. 2007. Policy design in strategic purchasing. In Preker AS, Liu X, Velenyi E, Baris E. (Editors). *Public Ends, Private Means: Strategic Purchasing of Health Services.* The International Bank for Reconstruction and Development. pp. 53–66.

[20] PPP Knowledge Lab. Health. https://pppknowledgelab.org/sectors/health. Accessed on January 30, 2021.

[21] Vian T, McIntosh N, Grabowski A. 2017. It keeps us from putting drugs in pockets: How a public-private partnership for hospital management may help curb corruption. *Permanente Journal.* 21: 16–113. http://www.thepermanente-journal.org/issues/2017/6469-"it-keeps-us-from-putting-drugs-in-pockets".html. Accessed on April 30, 2021.

Chapter 4

Malaria Medicines, Markets, and Public Policy

"They, and many others are asking now, in what world does it make sense to abandon a simple program that saves lives?"

—Kenneth J. Arrow[a]

"Until the lions have their own historians, the history of the hunt will always glorify the hunter."

—Chinua Achebe[b]

Synopsis

This chapter is an exploration of the conceptual origin, design, implementation, governance, and lessons learned from the Affordable Medicines Facility for Malaria (AMFm), with emphasis on the political economy of decision making around findings from its independent evaluation. Its first two sections draw upon the literature, especially but not only Frost and

---

[a]Arrow K. Saving a program that saves lives. *New York Times*. November 13, 2012. http://www.nytimes.com/2012/11/14/opinion/saving-a-malaria-program-that-saves-lives.html?_r=0. Accessed on December 20, 2020.

[b]Brooks J. 1994. Chinua Achebe, The Art of Fiction No. 139. *The Paris Review*. https://www.theparisreview.org/interviews/1720/the-art-of-fiction-no-139-chinua-achebe. Accessed on May 29, 2021.

Reich's report on the origins of what became the AMFm.[1-3] It gives the reader a driver's seat perspective of the dynamics of a disruptive innovation in global health. The chapter highlights the failures of the legacy architecture of development assistance for health, including how the United States Agency for International Development (USAID) and United States President's Malaria Initiative (US-PMI, an initiative led by USAID) undermined the health interests of the poor in countries that USAID and US-PMI claimed to serve.[c] It recalls published evidence of the empirical success of the AMFm. It examines the strategic failure of the Global Fund Board, lessons learned, the potential applicability of the private–public approach to other health commodities and countries, and the implications of this experience for evidence-based decisions in global health and development assistance.

4.1. The Context

Access to life-saving medicines and technologies was challenging at the beginning of the 21st century in many LICs and LMICs.[1] The reasons were multiple, including insufficient domestic health financing for drug purchases, weaknesses in supply chains, inappropriate prescriptions by service providers, and poor compliance by patients. These challenges played out in the context of long-standing debates about the roles of markets and the state in the health sector. Many countries took a government-run approach to the procurement and distribution of essential medicines, including centralized medical stores. Yet, there were government failures in the health sector too. This case study is situated against the background of trade-offs between market failures and government failures. How do the dynamics play out in practice?

In July 2004, I received a prepublication copy of a report by the Institute of Medicine (IOM) of the National Academies, entitled *Saving Lives, Buying Time: Economics of Malaria Drugs in an Age of*

---

[c]According to the US-PMI website, PMI is an interagency initiative led by the U.S. Agency for International Development (USAID) and implemented together with the U.S. Centers for Disease Control and Prevention (CDC). https://www.pmi.gov/about. Accessed on June 9, 2021.

Resistance.[4] Kenneth Arrow, a professor of economics and Nobel laureate, chaired the IOM panel that prepared the report. The report reached me on a hot and humid summer day of the sort that is familiar to those who grew up or lived in malaria-endemic tropical regions. But I had no idea of what it would unleash. I was literally about to leave for a vacation and my family had just arrived outside the office building to pick me up for a road trip, so I put it in my bag and left the office. A few days later, I read the report and realized that it was extraordinarily far-sighted, with a potential to make lives better for millions of malaria-afflicted people. As Coordinator of Public Health Programs at the World Bank and Chair of the Roll Back Malaria (RBM) Partnership's Working Group on Finance and Resources (RBM FRWG) at the time, I thought it was a rare opportunity to mobilize a potentially game-changing collective effort against a deadly foe: malaria was — and remains — a threat to lives and livelihoods in many parts of the world, especially but not only in Africa. The laid-back mode of downtime changed when I read that report. The first lesson from this chapter is to be careful what you read while on vacation.

4.2. Saving Lives, Buying Time

Saving Lives, Buying Time proposed a subsidy at the top of the global supply chain for a new generation of antimalarial medicines, the artemisinin-based combination treatments (ACTs). The WHO had recommended ACTs for the treatment of uncomplicated malaria caused by the parasite called *Plasmodium falciparum.*[5] The ACTs would replace the older medicines that were increasingly ineffective, such as chloroquine (CQ) and sulfadoxine-pyrimethamine (SP). But the causes of problems in accessing effective malaria treatments were multiple, and WHO's recommendation, while fundamental, would not solve two other problems.[2] First, DAH for malaria control was typically routed through the public sector, whereas people suffering from malaria mostly sought treatment in the private sector. The proposed subsidy would include the private sector and would benefit the public sector. Second, the new ACTs were very expensive compared to the failing CQ and SP; many who needed the ACTs could not easily afford to pay for them. In that context, the use of oral artemisinin monotherapy (AMT), which was cheaper than the ACTs, increased the risk of widespread resistance of the malaria parasite to artemisinin, which at the time was the only first-line treatment that remained widely effective. The proposed subsidy would reduce the cost of malaria medicines to people at the community level.

The proposal in *Saving Lives, Buying Time* was both ingenious and — I thought — doable. In one stroke, it would tackle the problem of affordability, reach those already being reached by existing outlets for the failing medicines, and help preserve the effectiveness of artemisinin for longer than would otherwise be the case.

Frost and colleagues wrote a substantive and insightful report[3] on the process of translating the concept proposed by *Saving Lives, Buying Time* into an implementable innovation called the Affordable Medicines Facility-malaria (AMFm). The reader will find that report and its associated teaching case[6] useful for a detailed understanding of the early dynamics that included multiple consultations by and across the RBM Partnership, representatives of malaria-endemic countries, WHO, GFATM, bilateral financiers, researchers, and many others, between 2004 and 2009.

It was at the Amsterdam Airport Schiphol, as we arrived for one of the many consultations, that I first met the late Kenneth Arrow. We were both waiting for our luggage at the carousel. An unusual weather pattern was causing flight delays in North America and Europe during that period. As we waited, he explained the links between weather patterns and decisions on flight delays. Having read about his wartime exploits in *Against The Gods*,[7] I knew that Arrow had a colorful history of engagement in weather forecasting. In measured and analytical terms, he gave me a masterclass on how air traffic controllers made decisions. We had many discussions in the following years and I learned a lot from him. Arrow often wondered how a simple idea of a global subsidy had become so complicated in the maze of the malaria world. Years later, one of our discussions lasted for about 90 minutes, ending around 10:30 pm in Geneva, where I was based (he was in California at the time). My son asked me what the long phone call was about and with whom, to which I responded, "That was Professor Arrow. We were discussing how a simple idea to get medicines to people with malaria has become very complicated. I have a lot of homework to do, just like you do." His eyes lit up: "Mom! Dad has homework!"

The early consultations resulted in a coalition that explored opportunities and options to translate *Saving Lives, Buying Time* into action. We started with no funds to work with. Faced with opposition to the global subsidy idea from within the World Bank's Development Economics Research Group (DEC), I invited Mead Over, the principal opponent of the global subsidy idea at DEC, to look into it with consultants of his choice. The RBM Secretariat, led by Professor Awa Coll-Seck, provided funds for the study. The study concluded as follows, first in a Research Working Paper and then in a peer-reviewed journal:[8]

> *"This study finds that a subsidy to ACTs is likely to slow the rate of emergence of resistance to artemisinin and partner drugs, even if such a subsidy were to increase the use of ACTs significantly. This conclusion is robust to alternative assumptions regarding the responsiveness of demand to the lower price for ACTs and a wide range of epidemiological and economic parameters."*

Based on that study, in July 2005 Francois Bourguignon (then Chief Economist and Senior Vice-President of DEC) and Jean-Louis Sarbib (then Senior Vice-President for Human Development) at the World Bank wrote to Arrow, noting the merit of *Saving Lives, Buying Time* and stating their interest in exploring its feasibility. At the Request of RBM, in 2005 the World Bank — as cochair of the RBM FRWG — agreed to formulate a proposal for the design and implementation of the global subsidy proposition. But there was a problem: the World Bank had no administrative budget for the design work. I teamed up with several colleagues including Andreas Seiter (a World Bank health specialist with prior experience in pharmaceutical industries), Ramanan Laxminarayan (then at Resources For the Future), and Hellen Gelband (study director of *Saving Lives, Buying Time*) to form a core group. On behalf of RBM, and with support from Girindre Beeharry and Daniel Kress of BMGF (both members of the RBM FRWG), the World Bank sought a grant from the BMGF to develop a plan that would translate the global subsidy from concept to action. The BMGF approved the grant in August 2006. At its meeting in Addis Ababa on November 29, 2007, the RBM Partnership Board approved further work to develop the AMFm.[9] The coalition had gained traction.

4.3. Innovation and Its Discontents

What followed was an intense and seemingly endless mix of seeking to advance science, translating a concept into an implementable program, building coalitions, navigating a minefield of entrenched and powerful guardians of the *status quo*, and enabling a shift in thinking and practice which, if it worked, would enormously benefit those being ravaged by malaria.

The process revolved around four objectives: developing a credible and viable architecture and plan to translate into practice the concepts proposed in *Saving Lives, Buying Time*; building a coalition to mobilize funds for the subsidy and political clout to secure global policy endorsement for a real-life test of concept; identifying and devising options to mitigate risks and potential derailers; and identifying options for hosting the subsidy mechanism. The grant from the BMGF funded the hiring of a consulting firm (Dalberg) and grant management expenses incurred by the World Bank, which set up a Project Management Team for the exercise.

The RBM Executive Committee endorsed the establishment of a Global ACT Subsidy Task Force (later renamed the AMFm Task Force), then charged it with building a consensus among RBM Partnership members on key dimensions of the global ACT subsidy and presenting its recommendations to the RBM Board. The cochairs of the Task Force were David Mwakyusa (Minister of Health of Tanzania) and Harry van Schooten (of the Netherlands Ministry of Foreign Affairs, representing Rob de Vos, an early supporter who departed to serve as the Dutch Ambassador to South Africa). John Worley of the U.K. DFID succeeded van Schooten on the Task Force at the end of 2007. The Task Force members included the BMGF, GFATM, NGOs, multilateral institutions like UNICEF, WHO, and the World Bank, bilateral entities like USAID, US-PMI, the private sector, academia and researchers, and several other RBM partners. Coll-Seck and her team at the RBM Secretariat supported the Task Force, for which the World Bank served as the hub through a subcontract with the consulting firm Dalberg.

4.3.1 Should it be considered at all?

The global subsidy idea shook up the hidebound and insular malaria control establishment. One very prominent opponent was Professor Richard Feachem, who was Executive Director of the GFATM at the time *Saving Lives, Buying Time* was published. He vehemently opposed the concept, and in an interview with Andrew Jack of the *Financial Times* in April 2007, Feachem said "It's not just getting the design right — we should not be doing it." (Box 4.1)

Box 4.1. Demonizing the Global Subsidy Proposal

- Sir Richard Feachem said the proposed subsidy risked failing those for whom it was intended and even worsening the incidence of malaria. He asserted that it would undermine pharmaceutical innovation and distract political commitment.
- Those comments came after a technical meeting that the Dutch government, which backed the subsidy proposal, hosted in Amsterdam.
- British officials had been involved in talks that could lead to a US$300 million annual subsidy to be launched in the following year.
- Professor Michel Kazatchkine, a French physician and AIDS expert, succeeded Sir Richard Feachem as Executive Director of the GFATM in April 2007.

Source: Jack A. 2007. Malaria Drug for the Poor 'a Bad Idea'. Financial Times. https://www.ft.com/content/36050d54-e6b3-11db-9034-000b5df 10621. Accessed on January 21, 2021.

On June 18, 2009, more than 2 years after the *Financial Times* publication, Feachem reached out to me. By then I was serving as founding director of the AMFm at the Global Fund. On behalf of his Global Health Group at the University of California in San Francisco, he sought collaboration around market-based malaria treatment and noted that this was an area where the Group's expertise and contacts could support the "terrific work" that my colleagues and I were setting out to do at the AMFm. He solicited a written note from me to indicate support for a proposal by his University of California group for a plan of work around market-based malaria treatment. It came across as seeking to quietly benefit from an enterprise that he had ruthlessly vilified in the public domain. Regardless, my duty called for laser-like focus on making the AMFm work and on learning from it. Therefore, I advised Feachem as follows:

> *"Relationships with the AMFm (planning and funding): The AMFm already has a business plan that includes several workstreams, of which operations research is a key component. It also has planned activities with multiple technical partners, in addition to the oversight mechanisms mandated by the Global Fund Board. Being a small team with a tight budget, we have neither the spare bandwidth nor extra funds to co-organize or co-finance the proposed Plan of Work. This constraint is much to my regret. But we have a keen interest in learning from the proposed exercise, and we would be much honored to learn from your team in particular.*
>
> *Specific considerations: Given the combination of real constraints and our team's interest in the substance of the work as noted above, I suggest that you kindly consider the following approach:*
>
> – *Regarding the proposed Country Case Studies and the Expert Group Meeting: Please plan this as an exercise that is independent of the AMFm. This is because the AMFm will neither provide an official endorsement for, nor cosponsor the Plan of Work. We will participate in major activities to which we are invited, with a view to learning and also contributing on the basis of early experiences from AMFm Phase 1.*
> – *Regarding the proposed Operations Research Studies: We are discussing with several partners some alternative approaches to operations research, with a view to agreeing on research questions and avoiding wasteful overlaps and gaps among the actors. We would be pleased to invite your team to join the discussion. If the discussions are successful, we would endorse a funding proposal from your team to potential financiers along the agreed lines.*
> – *Regarding the proposed dissemination of publications: Our interests are to see peer-reviewed publications in the public domain and to make them available to those who will conduct the independent*

evaluation of AMFm Phase 1. I believe that these are well aligned with the proposal."

Feachem and I kept in touch, on and off, during the AMFm, and within the parameters indicated above, I engaged in some ways with his group.

Feachem's early and vehement opposition was understandable. He was heading the GFATM and here was a disruptive innovation that might take the sheen off the GFATM's comparatively ossified and conventional approach to financing and enabling access to malaria medicines. But while it was understandable, it was also misguided. He could have engaged with the RBM Partnership and sought to test the proposition as a potential business window of the GFATM, thus giving the GFATM an opportunity to spearhead a new way of doing business. His subsequent acknowledgment of the "terrific work" would have been noble if it had been done as publicly as the strident condemnation in the *Financial Times*.

The lesson here is the need for leaders in global health to avoid the misstep of hastily condemning and dismissing new ideas that did not originate from them. The perils of hasty and unwise condemnation are illustrated by the mistake of Linus Pauling, the exceptional scientist who was awarded two individual Nobel Prizes (one for Chemistry, the other for Peace),[10] yet closed his mind to the spectacular discovery of the structure of quasicrystals by his supervisee Dan Shechtman, who went on to win a Nobel Prize for that discovery.[11]

4.3.2　USAID versus Africans: Of primetime and watches

The US President's Malaria Initiative (US-PMI) was the richest, most powerful, and most ruthless opponent of the AMFm. They weaponized their clout against the global subsidy proposition. To understand the origin and effects of their stance and actions, it is important to go back in time. Two years before the publication of *Saving Lives, Buying Time*, the *New York Times* had reported on USAID opposition to ensuring the availability of artemisinin in Africa. Their reason reportedly included high costs and a belief that the drug would be hard for poor people to take correctly. The

New York Times also reported that USAID quietly pressured African country officials not to even request artemisinin (Box 4.2).

Box 4.2. How USAID Slow-Walked New Malaria Drug in Africa

- 2,000 African children were dying of malaria every day.
- Doctors in Africa sought to use the new drug called artemisinin. Dr. David Nabarro, executive director in the office of WHO's Executive Director, said "It really is a marvelous drug."
- The United States opposed the use of artemisinin in Africa at that time.
- Dr. Dennis Carroll of the USAID reportedly said the medicine represented "the best long-term solution." He added that the drug was expensive and hard for poorly educated people to take correctly. Dr. Carroll reportedly asserted that the medicine was "not ready for prime time."
- Some African public health officers complained that USAID pressured them not to even request artemisinin.
- Dr. Rosemary Sunkutu, the public health director in Zambia, said the American Embassy's aid representative in Lusaka asked her to keep using the cheaper drugs (i.e., the failing drugs).
- Dr. Fred Binka, a professor of epidemiology at the University of Ghana, said "If you had such resistance levels to a drug in the West, you know there would be an outcry."

Source: McNeil DG. 2002. New Drug for Malaria Pits US against Africa. https://www.nytimes.com/2002/05/28/health/new-drug-for-malaria-pits-us-against-africa.html. Accessed on January 21, 2021.

The belief that artemisinin would be hard for poor people to take correctly was not based on credible science. It was part of a narrative marinated in structural racism, as was an assertion by Andrew Natsios, a former Administrator of USAID:

"Many Africans don't know what Western time is," he told the Boston Globe. "You have to take these (AIDS) drugs a certain number of hours

a day, or they don't work. Many people in Africa have never seen a clock or a watch their entire lives. They know morning, they know noon, they know evening, they know the darkness at night."[12]

The published record of Natsios's 2001 testimony to the United States Congress includes the following:

"So the biggest problem, if you look at Kofi Annan's budget, half the budget is for antiretrovirals. If we had them today, we could not distribute them. We could not administer the program because we do not have the doctors, the roads, we do not have the cold chain. This sounds small and some people, if you have traveled to rural Africa you know this, this is not a criticism, just a different world. People do not know what watches and clocks are. They do not use western means for telling time. They use the sun. These drugs have to be administered during a certain sequence of time during the day and when you say take at 10:00, people will say what do you mean by 10:00? They do not use those terms in the villages to describe the morning and afternoon and the evening. So that is a problem."[13]

The United States of America embodies an essential goodness and an extraordinary greatness. However, fountains of toxic ignorance and purveyors of racialist narratives are fetid sores on that essential goodness. Natsios's statement was astonishing in its idiocy, but that was not the fundamental problem, given that the United States Capitol had seen ignorami before that episode. The exemplar of such performances was that of William P. Clark, whom President Ronald Reagan nominated to be his Deputy Secretary of State in 1981. So extreme was Clark's display of ignorance of foreign affairs at the Senate Foreign Relations Committee hearings that *Newsweek* labelled him *A Truly Open Mind.*[14] In fairness to Clark, he admitted the exceptional modesty of his knowledge. By contrast, Natsios's claim came across as galling in its smug arrogance, evil in its cruelty, and dangerous in its lack of empirical basis with reference to adherence to AIDS treatment. There is evidence, from systematic review and meta-analysis, of higher adherence to treatment among Africans than among North Americans.[15] One study found "highest levels of complete adherence in Latin America (89%) and Africa (73%) and lowest levels in North America (45%; $P < .05$ comparing Africa and Brazil to any other region)."[16]

The *New York Times* report and the Congressional testimony were among the publicly known positions of USAID officials on whether or not Africans should have access to new and effective medicines for treating malaria and AIDS, respectively, well before the IOM published *Saving Lives, Buying Time* in 2004. The pronouncements were worthy of Edgar Rice Burroughs, who based his adventure fantasy on a continent about which he was utterly ignorant, but nevertheless found a ready audience for stories based on *Tarzan of the Apes*.[17] It is remarkable that life was imitating art of the vile variety in that testimony. But it was not an original sin. Ronald Reagan was on tape with the following statement about African diplomats to the United Nations:

> *"To watch that thing on television, as I did, to see those, those monkeys from those African countries — damn them, they're still uncomfortable wearing shoes!" Reagan tells Nixon, who erupts in laughter.*[18,19]

Those familiar with the dog whistles and tropes of racism in the domestic politics of the United States will recall the nefarious doctrine of Lee Atwater:[20]

> *"You start out in 1954 by saying, "Nigger, nigger, nigger." By 1968 you can't say "nigger" — that hurts you. Backfires. So you say stuff like forced busing, states' rights and stuff like that."*

Reflecting on the toxic racism of former US Presidents Richard Nixon and Ronald Reagan, the historian Tim Naftali noted the foreign policy ramifications of bigoted leadership:[21]

> *"Nixon's comments don't come as a surprise to me. Reagan's comment did. Nixon's comments are worth learning about today as a reminder that when people with power express bigoted ideas, not only are those words bad, but they have a meaning and a significance that is much bigger than one would assume. Richard Nixon made clear to Daniel*

Patrick Moynihan that his sense that African Americans and Africans were inferior would shape his welfare policies. And Richard Nixon makes clear on the tapes that his dislike of African leaders will shape the way in which he interacts with them in terms of foreign policy. So that means that bigotry shaped Nixon's domestic and foreign policy. In this era, when we have a head of state who uses racially charged — and I would say, most recently, racist terms and tweets — we have to keep in mind that this is not just a matter of one man's flaws. This may be injecting poison into the decisions that this administration is making on foreign and domestic issues. That's why revisiting the Nixon tapes and learning what is new on them is of real importance today."

Unwittingly, perhaps, USAID was channeling into the global arena the racist tropes deployed by some leaders in domestic United States politics. It might no longer be fashionable to call Africans "monkeys," but it was acceptable to use dog whistles about Africans not knowing what time it was. Twenty years after the toxic testimony of Natsios, the United States Centers for Disease Control and Prevention (US-CDC) "declared racism a public health threat."[22] That was with reference to structural racism. To heal the open sores on the essential goodness of the United States, the US-CDC might do the world a service by educating and nudging USAID and US-PMI into the 21st century on matters of racist narratives in global health. It is past time to overhaul a foreign aid model that is predicated on racist tropes.

In sum, when *Saving Lives, Buying Time* was published, USAID did nothing to take the idea forward. Its subsequent approach was a combination of hostility and plausible deniability via obfuscation. All were harbingers of what US-PMI would later do to the AMFm. As for Africa, the natives couldn't possibly run private sector supply chains to deliver ACTs, could they? It was evocative of *Tarzan of the Apes*, who dearly loved and understood the shoeless and watchless *natives*, thus legitimizing for US-PMI the sole capacity and exclusive rights to think for, speak for, and do the job for them.

It is cosmically fitting that USAID is headquartered in the Ronald Reagan Building and International Trade Center on Pennsylvania Avenue in Washington DC. Would-be saviors of Africans might be forgiven for taking a Reaganesque doctrine if, on the way to the continent, they exited the Ronald Reagan Building, saw the Ronald Reagan statue as they approached the Ronald Reagan Airport, then jetted off to talk sense to the watchless *natives*.

4.4. Will It Work?

The global subsidy was conceptually brilliant and path breaking, but whether it would work in practice was an open question. Nobody in global health had ever tried it before. It flew in the face of traditional practices in getting malaria medicines to patients. The major questions that the RBM Global Subsidy Task Force and the World Bank Team sought to answer during the design period included the following:

(a) Would manufacturers of ACTs even agree to negotiate prices with a global subsidy entity?

(b) Would those same manufacturers agree to comply with WHO Guidelines against AMTs?

(c) What would be the appropriate levels of subsidies, and how would they be determined?

(d) Would "middlemen" — the private sector importers, distributors, and retailers — in participating countries charge exorbitant mark-ups, thus gouging the market and preventing the subsidy from being passed on to the patients who would purchase ACTs at the retail outlets? This was at the core of an anticipated shift from low volumes with high margins to high volumes with low margins.

(e) How would ACTs under the global subsidy be distinguished from other ACTs?

(f) Would the subsidized ACTs reach rural populations and those far from major commercial hubs? This was going to be a test of the effectiveness of domestic private sector supply chains in participating countries. In the political economy of DAH, if the global subsidy succeeded by using the local supply chains, it would pose an existential threat to those legacy business models of foreign aid that were based upon channeling large sums of money to foreign contractors who would then set up their own supply chains to distribute medicines in developing countries. USAID and US-PMI's business model was at risk of extinction.

(g) How would the needs of both the public sector and private sector pharmacies be met?

(h) Would there be timely and sufficient quantities of *Artemisia annua*, the plant from which artemisinin was derived?

(i) How would the evolution of the ACT market be tracked during implementation?

(j) Given the aversion in some quarters to the word "subsidy," what would the global subsidy mechanism be called? Many in the public health field had for long worked on malaria but were not versed in the economic concepts of public goods (i.e., nonrivalry and nonexcludability), externalities, and business economics. How might their comfort level be increased? Following multiple consultations with stakeholders, Coll-Seck (Executive Director of RBM) and I jointly decided on the name "Affordable Medicines Facility for malaria (AMFm)."

(k) Would massive quantities of subsidized ACTs under the AMFm be diverted to neighboring non-AMFm countries for excessive profit? The issue here was not to seek perfection; anyone working in LICs and MICs would not expect absolutely zero leakage across borders if there were huge price differences. Afterall, there was cross-border price arbitrage of medicines from Canada to the United States. Surely the solution there was not to abolish the system that enabled Canadians to access essential medicines at much lower prices than their southern neighbors?[23] Furthermore, if the ultimate biological benefit accrued to a person who would otherwise have had no ACT, and reduced the likelihood of malaria parasite transmission to others, was that inherently bad? What economic incentives might be appropriate to deter such cross-border arbitrage in LIC and LMIC settings? Was the solution to have no subsidized medicines, or to have subsidized medicines everywhere, or rely on the wishful thinking of command-and-control methods that would not work at the Canada–USA border, hence no chance of working at the very porous borders of many LICs and LMICs? What might be the least-bad attainable options from a very practical perspective?

(1) How could the known opponents of the AMFm (such as the US-PMI) be reassured that the innovation was truly an exploration subject to empirical test? The solution to this was to call the pilot phase AMFm Phase 1. Any subsequent phase would objectively consider the results from Phase 1. Even this solution was unsatisfactory to some, on the basis that it signaled a progression to Phase 2. What was under-appreciated was the extent to which opposition to Phase 1 itself was so averse to any evidence that no amount of evidence would change the minds of the AMFm's opponents, especially the US-PMI.

In November 2007, the AMFm Task Force of the RBM Partnership published the technical design of the AMFm, which provided initial answers to many of the design questions and opened up the possibility of testing their feasibility through large, country-wide pilots in a first phase.[24]

The design of AMFm included three key parts: price reductions through negotiations with manufacturers of ACTs; a buyer subsidy, via a copayment at the top of the global supply chain; and support of interventions to promote appropriate use of ACTs. One key innovation was the combination of price reductions through negotiations with manufacturers and a global subsidy. The subsidy was done in the form of copayment by the AMFm of a substantial part of the post-negotiation price. Eligible first-line buyers (from the public sector, the private sector, and NGOs), who purchased quality-assured ACTs directly from the manufacturers, would pay the modest remainder of the post-negotiation price. The other key innovation, which was not a headliner but was a potential disruptor of the *status quo* in development assistance for malaria medicines, was the explicit use of in-country private sector supply chains and outlets. That would effectively bypass large foreign firms contracted by any bilateral or multilateral financier to undertake supply chain management and distribution of malaria medicines. Therefore, it was a threat to that long-entrenched business model.

By aiming to reduce the cost of ACTs sold in private sector outlets from up to US$11 per treatment in 2010, to the same price as CQ and SP (about US$0.50) and to less than the cost of oral AMT (about US$3–7), the AMFm was a potentially transformative business model. Those seeking malaria treatment at public health centers or NGO facilities would also benefit from better access to more affordable or free-of-charge ACTs in those settings.

In September 2009, the report of a small pilot study within Tanzania, which was funded by the BMGF, indicated that the basic design of subsidized ACT worked at the subnational level. Sabot and colleagues concluded as follows:[25]

> "A subsidy introduced at the top of the private sector supply chain can significantly increase usage of ACTs and reduce their retail price to the level of common monotherapies. Additional interventions may be needed to ensure access to ACTs in remote areas and for poorer individuals who appear to seek treatment at drug shops less frequently."

4.5. Hosting and Financing

What kind of hosting arrangement would be most suitable and which institution would host the first phase of the AMFm? Multiple options were considered. The GFATM seemed like the most appropriate option, given its stated committed to innovation and status as a public–private partnership dedicated to fighting AIDS, TB, and malaria. However, the GFATM's *de facto* understanding and comfort zone of public–private engagement before the spring of 2007 was to raise funds from the private sector and spend it via grants to public sector entities and not-for-profit private entities. Spending money through the commercial private sector to achieve public policy goals was not in the comfort zone of GFATM at the time. That changed in 2007, when Kazatchkine succeeded Feachem as Executive Director of GFATM. Kazatchkine was open to the proposal in *Saving Lives, Buying Time*, asked tough questions about its feasibility — directly and via his adviser Jean-Paul Moatti (an economist), and was a force for thoughtful inquiry in his engagement with the RBM Partnership, the Task Force, and the World Bank's team. That engagement paved the way for the RBM Board to consider inviting the GFATM to host the AMFm. The RBM Board, at its meeting on November 28–29, 2007, invited the GFATM to host and manage the AMFm.

The GFATM Board met in New Delhi on November 7–8, 2008. That was its 18th meeting, and the agenda included a decision on whether to host and manage the global ACT subsidy for an initial phase in a limited number of countries.[26] The prospects for start-up funding from financiers other than the GFATM were positive. By the beginning of 2009, funding commitments had been secured from two financiers — DFID and the new entity called UNITAID, providing enough funding to start AMFm Phase 1. A few other key financiers — the BMGF and the Government of Canada — would later commit funds.

That GFATM Board Meeting was held in the wake of Barack Obama's spectacular ascent to the presidency of the United States. The humanity and riveting campaign of the preceding weeks were unprecedented. On the eve of the election, I had a memorable discussion with a gentleman who was a security guard in the office building where I worked in Washington DC, across the street from the White House complex. This tall, middle-aged gentleman was of Caribbean origin. We would greet each other every day but he usually was a man of few words and no banter. Something different happened on that day. I said "good morning, sir" to him and turned slightly to go to the elevator. He responded in a booming, yet silky baritone:

"Good morning. It's gonna be a big day tomorrow. Win or lose, I'm gonna cry, because I'm so proud of him."

I froze. When I turned around to look at him, this normally imperturbable man had tears in his eyes. It all hit home. A man who shared his skin color just might become President of the United States. Before I knew it, I was reaching for tissue to dry my eyes. Yes, a man who shared my young sons' skin color was on the cusp of doing the seemingly impossible. Sometimes, life is positively magical. The drive home on election day was surreal as the polls were about to close on the east coast of the United

States. Crowds were gathering at street junctions along the main artery of Connecticut Avenue. Strangers were hugging. Drivers were honking auditory signals that the improbable was about to happen. In a call-and-response rhythm of communal joy, a pedestrian would give a thumbs up and drivers would honk three times as other pedestrians chanted in sync: *O-ba-ma!*

I left Washington DC for New Delhi on the day after the election of Barack Obama. There was a joyful buzz all around. The German passenger sitting next to me on the flight from Washington DC to Frankfurt that night wanted to do nothing but seek my perspectives on everything Obama, so there was no sleeping on that transatlantic leg of the trip. The security agent at the gate check in Frankfurt, unprompted, asked me to take the red-carpet lane, offered congratulations, and gave a foot-wide smile. What had they just started smoking in Frankfurt-am-Main? I was used to getting extra scrutiny and had once been detained for hours by a Frankfurt airport official who, despite written evidence, just would not believe that I was indeed going to a scientific conference, until his supervisor's supervisor set him straight and apologized to "Herr Doktor Doktor." This brown skin was suddenly talismanic! On arrival at night in New Delhi, the cab driver congratulated me on the great Obama victory: "India has Gandhi, now America has Obama." The usually staid bureaucrats at the GFATM Board meeting even loosened up and spent minutes watching and laughing at the endlessly looping Tom and Jerry cartoons on small video screens near the hotel's elevators. One could almost touch the positivity in the air. Bless you, President-elect Obama!

Despite years of work and months of specific preparation for a Board decision on hosting, led by the Policy and Strategy (PSC) Committee of the GFATM Board, the outcome was dicey. The GFATM Board discussion of whether to host the AMFm was not straightforward. It was a mini opera in which key actors were prepositioning for their next acts. The US delegation worked against the AMFm. It portrayed itself as the entity with a monopoly of wisdom on which innovation was worth exploring and was clear that the AMFm was not worth exploring. The following record of the proceedings gives a glimpse of what transpired (Box 4.3), but did not fully convey the breadth, ruthlessness, and relentlessness of the US delegation's scheming behind the scenes.

Box 4.3. Discussion of the AMFm at the GFATM Board Meeting, November 2008

4. "The (Policy and Strategy Committee) PSC presentation continued the next morning with a presentation of the decision point on the AMFm. The PSC Chair said that a number of consultations had taken place since the Sixteenth Board Meeting and that the PSC has had a long debate about the subject as well. He was happy that the PSC was able to come to consensus on a decision point about the issue.

5. A number of delegates indicated their strong support for the initiative due to the increased opportunities it provided to get effective drugs to the poor and into rural areas, as well as its public private partnership model. However, it was also highlighted the AMFm may be difficult to manage and that care needed to be taken to ensure that the AMFm did not crowd out other Global Fund initiatives, and that the AMFm could effectively be adapted to the Global Fund business model. On this issue several delegates questioned whether the AMFm was an appropriate business line for the Global Fund and if the initiative should not be hosted and managed elsewhere.

6. The Point Seven delegation acknowledged that while taking on a new business line involves risk, there is also risk involved with not pursuing the AMFm as it is a way to have real impact on malaria by increasing access to drugs. The delegation felt that the Global Fund has a lot of responsibility in this instance and saw the discussion as one that is related to the discussion on the Global Fund's role as an investor in malaria.

7. While reiterating that universal access is a goal of the Board, the delegation from the United States (US) said that it differed in its views on how to achieve that. The US delegation outlined several concerns with the AMFm: Whether it is appropriate for the Global Fund and whether it is workable or feasible at all. The delegation believes that the proposal is inconsistent with the Global Fund's mission and implored the Board to have the courage to recognize when a big new idea is not a good one.

    The delegation said it would like to continue to work over the next six months to address the following issues: expansion of access to the poorest of the poor; a clear comparison between value for money and other potential models for access to treatment in terms of reduction of mortality; safety concerns with regard to pregnant women and children with fevers; implications for changes to the Global Fund business model, framework, and technical processes; the makeup of an independent technical body; and valid criteria for applications. Given these concerns, the delegation asked that the decision point include the word exploratory instead of transitional when describing the AMFm Committee.

8. The WHO delegation cautioned the Board that it is very important to get the technical aspects of the AMFm right from the beginning, especially in terms of policies regarding the administration of drugs to children with fevers and steps that should be taken to prevent drug resistance.

9. The Developed Country NGO delegation expressed deep concern about issues regarding safety — especially in light of the problems that arose because of over- and under-prescription of chloroquine which is no longer a useful treatment option. The delegation also said that it sees distribution of free bed net and free ACTs as very useful, especially because women and children are largely affected.

10. Due to the concerns raised it was suggested that the AMFm be introduced in a phased approach and that it be kept under review by both the PSC and the Board.

11. In preparation for the vote on the decision point, the PSC Chair said he believed the decision point invited the opportunity for the Board to express its concerns. He proposed that the committee referred to in the decision point be called an ad hoc committee. The decision point passed. The Board Chair noted that Japan did not vote."

Source: GFATM. *Eighteenth Board Meeting GF/B18/2.* New Delhi, India, November 7–8, 2008. Pages 17–18. https://www.theglobalfund.org/board-decisions/b18-dp03/. Accessed on January 25, 2021.

Finally, the GFATM Board agreed to have the GFATM Secretariat prepare to host and manage the AMFm as a business line within the Global Fund. The Secretariat would do so in consultation with the RBM Partnership and all relevant stakeholders. The GFATM Board established the AMFm Ad-hoc Committee of the Board to oversee and guide the work. It specifically noted that "Membership of the AMFm Ad-hoc

Committee shall not apply towards the two-committee limit set out in Section 23 of the Board Operating Procedures."

The GFATM Board decision marked the end of the initial phase of translating the *Saving Lives, Buying Time* report into an implementable program design. There remained operational details to be defined. Those would be done during the period between the Board Meeting and the formal launch of AMFm in April 2009.

I called home to give my family the good news of the decision by the GFATM Board. It had been a long and intense haul since that hot summer day in 2004 and the GFATM would now take on the implementation of AMFm Phase 1. I could concentrate on my work programs at the World Bank. Then Kazatchkine asked me: with the Board approval, the GFATM Secretariat now had to test the AMFm innovation in practice — would I lead the big experiment? Four months later, with a deep sense of duty and curiosity about what we might achieve and learn, I moved to Geneva as founding director of the AMFm at the GFATM on time-bound leave from the World Bank. There was a lot of learning ahead at the frontiers of markets and public policy for improved access to malaria medicines.

4.6. Implementation: Joys of Learning and Perils of Intrigue

"… I knew that I was walking in a field strewn with dangerous, explosive mines where one false step might signal my demise. What was surprising were depths of intrigue, scheming, conspiracy, and maneuvering."

—Adetokunbo Lucas[d]

4.6.1 Launch and implementation

The formal and public launch of the AMFm was held in April 2009 in Oslo, Norway. Several stakeholders noted the possibilities of the initiative. For example:[27]

---

[d]Lucas AO. 2010. *It Was the Best of Times: From Local to Global Health.* Ibadan, Nigeria: BookBuilders. p. 175.

"The age when the world had effective drugs against infectious diseases but let millions die each year because they couldn't afford them is over," said Foreign Minister Jonas Gahr Støre of Norway, "Thanks to new commitments, collaboration, and finance build up over the last decade, we are making these deaths history. The results will go beyond saving lives: malaria is costing developing countries billions of dollars each year in lost economic output. By controlling malaria, we can improve school attendance and productivity, open new areas to business and tourism and reduce health costs."

"This partnership is an important part of the global effort to control malaria worldwide," said Dr Michel Kazatchkine, Executive Director of the Global Fund. "There is no reason any child should die of malaria anymore. We have insecticide-impregnated bed nets to protect families from mosquitoes and effective drugs to treat those who do fall ill. Now we only need to ensure that all who need these things get them. This is a very wise investment in global health — and therefore in global development."

"The Affordable Medicines Facility for malaria is a breakthrough in global health," said Robert B. Zoellick, President of the World Bank Group. "It will help to treat the millions of people who suffer from malaria illness and death every year and prolong the effectiveness of new anti-malarial medicines. It is a striking example of partnerships that really work. We are pleased the World Bank Group could help create and support the new Facility, and we are appreciative that the Global Fund will now lead its implementation."

"We are proud that the Netherlands was a key partner during the early stages of the Affordable Medicines Facility for malaria's design and development, and we are impressed with the outcomes of this collaborative process," said Netherlands Minister for Development Cooperation Bert Koenders. "We warmly welcome the contributions already pledged by UNITAID and the United Kingdom, and are pleased to announce that the Netherlands is also considering a financial contribution to the AMFm."

"What we are doing is using market dynamics to save more lives," said Dr Philippe Douste-Blazy, Chairman of the board of UNITAID. "Through the provision of predictable funding, manufacturers will see an incentive to bring prices down and new producers will be motivated to enter the market. The result: better medicines available to millions of women and children."

"Every year nearly one million people living in developing countries die from malaria — that's around 2,500 people a day," said the UK International Development Minister, Ivan Lewis. "The Affordable Medicines Facility for Malaria could save up to 300,000 lives every year — mostly children's — by making the best treatments available at affordable prices. That is why the UK has been a driving force behind the initiative and why we stand ready to support all efforts to reduce the unacceptable human burden of this disease."

"The Affordable Medicines Facility for malaria is a triumph of international cooperation," said Prof Awa-Marie Coll-Seck, Executive Director of the RBM Partnership. "This initiative responds to the current and urgent need to get more effective malaria medicines to where they are needed most. The roll out of the AMFm in coming months will contribute to our collective goal of universal access and to improving maternal and child health worldwide."

"The Affordable Medicines Facility for malaria is an exciting effort to improve access to life-saving malaria drugs, and to replace old drugs that are no longer as effective as they once were," said Dr Tachi Yamada, President of the Bill & Melinda Gates Foundation Global Health Program. "This is an important part of a broader effort to prevent and treat malaria, and reduce substantially the terrible toll that this disease takes on so many."

News reports of the launch in the *New York Times* quoted the Deputy Coordinator of the US-PMI as deriding the AMFm as "the biggest faith-based initiative in the world of malaria."[28] That quote in the *New York Times* was representative of US-PMI's boorish arrogance and contempt for learning.

A small group that included Christina Schrade and Andrew Freeman had worked with the GFATM's Executive Director's office and liaised with the Dalberg team to prepare for the GFTAM Board's consideration of the hosting decision and to explore workstreams that would be developed during implementation. Following the decision by the GFATM Board, a lean and dedicated team managed the implementation of AMFm Phase 1 at the GFATM Secretariat in Geneva. Andrew Freeman, Martine Donoghue, Fabienne Jouberton, and Margot Morris worked long hours and were collectively effective as we built the program in those early days. We were later joined by Emmanuel Yuniwo Nfor, Esther Otieno, David

Eastman, Nana Boohene, Melisse Murray, Silas Holland, Werner Buhler, Lloyd Matowe, and Toyin Jolayemi. The AMFm team worked with and through multiple departments of the GFATM Secretariat to avoid creating needless duplications and to promote what Michel Kazatchkine often called "transversal" approaches in the Secretariat.

The transversal approach worked most of the time, and it sometimes worked excellently. Among the most professional and dedicated GFATM senior managers who contributed significantly to the AMFm were Rifat Atun (Director of the Strategy, Performance, and Evaluation Cluster), Gulen Newton (General Counsel, Legal Department), Edward Addai (Director, Monitoring and Evaluation), Fareed Abdullah (Africa Unit Director, who went on to lead the South African National AIDS Council), Will Ashby (Director of Procurement), Orion Yeandel (Contract Specialist), Josephine Mbithi (Human Resources), and Jon Liden (Communications Director). They had positive influence on many staff members, including several Fund Portfolio Managers with whom the AMFm Team engaged. Many GFATM staff members, especially but not only those who were well aware of the limitations of the GFATM's traditional grant model, saw merit in testing how well the AMFm might work. Most were positively curious about it. However, there remained pockets of hostility to the AMFm, carried over from the days of Professor Richard Feachem. They were ardent practitioners of intrigue, scheming, turfism, pettiness, and — worst of all — aversion to learning. In April 2009, one senior adviser brought out a pile of papers on the global subsidy idea, dumped them on the table, asked me to take them away as if ridding himself of a vial of the plague bacterium, and gleefully proclaimed: "it can never work!" A senior manager in the pharmaceuticals unit seemingly delighted in gumming up the works of anything related to the AMFm.

There were three main workstreams at the start of the AMFm, all of which were overseen by the AMFm Ad Hoc Committee of the GFATM Board:

- Country Access and Applications;
- Copayment Strategy and Negotiations With Manufacturers, which included the Clinton Health Access Initiative (CHAI) as Negotiation Agent; and

- Monitoring and Evaluation (covering the commissioning of an independent evaluation, in consultation with the GFATM's Technical Evaluation Reference Group and an independent expert group for advice on methods for the independent evaluation).[29]

The evolution of the work programs led to their modifications and the additions of workstreams in market dynamics, supply chain management, and operations and coordination, with team members working in overlapping groups that enabled rapid and effective communication across workstreams.

The AMFm team performed and/or commissioned activities, and coconvened forums that achieved the following mission-critical steps during implementation:

(a) ACT price negotiations with manufacturers of WHO-prequalified ACTs: These covered ACTs that met the AMFm's requirements, based on WHO guidelines and prequalification standards.

(b) Master Supply Agreements with ACT manufacturers, including Ajanta Pharma, Cipla, Guilin Pharmaceuticals, Ipca Laboratories, Novartis, and Sanofi-Aventis. The agreements slashed the manufacturer price for sales to private sector purchasers by a range (about 29–78%), down to about the same as for public sector buyers.[30]

(c) Definition and agreement on a factory-gate buyer subsidy (the AMFm co-payment): This included subsidy levels for different product types and formulations. A Co-payment Technical Advisory Group, ably chaired by Professor Prashant Yadav, provided very sensible advice that informed the AMFm's decisions.

(d) Request for applications to participate in the AMFm, including the private and public sector of countries included in Phase 1.

(e) Branding of AMFm copaid ACT packs via a Green Leaf logo. This was an exercise in branding and marketing. Penny Grewal of the Medicines for Malaria Ventures made excellent contributions to this exercise, both in substance and in effective coalition building with multiple actors that included CHAI.

(f) Payment by AMFm of a substantial portion of the post-negotiation price. This was the "copayment" on behalf of eligible first-line buyers from the public and private sectors and NGOs, who all purchased quality-assured ACTs directly from the manufacturers. The AMFm did not play the role of a procurement agent. The ACT importers paid manufacturers a subsidized price of about 1–20% of the manufacturer price. The AMFm copayment fund paid the balance.

(g) Definition of a suite of supporting interventions: These included public information, advertisements, price ceiling recommendations, and guidelines that were developed within participating countries.

Following the preparations noted above, Phase one of AMFm started in mid-2010 and it lasted for 2 years. It was planned for implementation in eight national-level pilots in Cambodia, Ghana, Kenya, Madagascar, Nigeria, Niger, Tanzania (including the mainland and Zanzibar), and Uganda. The period covered by the independent evaluation was much less than 2 years because the *effective implementation period* was from the time the first subsidized ACTs arrived in each country until data were collected for the evaluation.

Other important activities included periodic market surveys to monitor early developments and trends in the market for ACTs in participating countries; applicable elements of pharmacovigilance, insofar as this was appropriate and feasible; and small-scale implementation research to inform program execution and fine-tuning.

4.6.2 It works!

Thursday, September 30, 2010, was a special day for the AMFm team. Lloyd Matowe, who combined conceptual heft with operational savvy, had visited Ghana and purchased a few packs of AMFm-branded ACTs. In Ghana, unlike the public sector, the private sector importers, also called the First-Line Buyers, had moved swiftly to register with the AMFm and then started importing the AMFm-branded ACTs. They were so effective that public sector managers in some districts of Ghana started purchasing their ACTs from the private sector distributors within the country. It was an indication of the relative ineffectiveness of the public sector as an importer and distributor of malaria medicines. Lloyd came straight from the airport to the office, brandishing the ACTs and grinning from ear to ear. At first, there was silence as the importance of the moment sank in: against all the odds, despite all the doubts, the AMFm had actually succeeded in getting those co-paid ACTs from the factory gate, through the local private sector supply chain, to the retail outlet in a peri-urban setting. Then the room erupted in cheers.

The team had expected it to work, but it was not a certainty. Now here was the empirical, physical proof. It was a moment of utter joy. Several team members dashed to the office of Kazatchkine on the next floor down and we interrupted his meeting by waving the ACT pack so that he could see it through the glass wall. He stood up, came out, and got the good news. Kazatchkine later recalled hearing two words over and over:

"It works! It works!! It works!!!"

This, to the team, was on a par with the first human landing on the moon. The Eagle had landed. But certain parties were hell-bent on ensuring that it never made it back to earth; if you cannot beat the achievement, shoot down the spacecraft and insist it never landed on the moon.

4.6.3 Oversight

GFATM Board oversight of the AMFm was vested in the AMFm Ad Hoc Committee (Box 4.4). It did much commendable work and also became a prime battleground between those who genuinely sought to guide a rigorous test of the AMFm on the one hand, and those who sought to destroy it on the other hand.

Box 4.4. AMFm Ad Hoc Committee Terms of Reference

The AMFm Ad Hoc Committee is an ad hoc committee of the Board established for the sole purpose of overseeing and advising the Board on the development, launch, implementation and evaluation of the first phase of the Affordable Medicines Facility for Malaria (AMFm).

(Continued)

Box 4.4. (*Continued*)

Terms of Reference

The committee shall have the following responsibilities:

- Oversee the preparations for launch of the AMFm Phase 1, review reports provided by the Secretariat and provide guidance to the Secretariat.
- Advise the Board on critical strategic and policy matters related to AMFm Phase 1.
- Provide regular updates to the Board on progress.
- Oversee the independent evaluation of AMFm Phase 1 and report the findings to the Board.
- Based on the results of the independent evaluation, make recommendations to the Board on whether to expand, accelerate, terminate or suspend the AMFm business line. In fulfilling these responsibilities the committee will have regard to the Principles for AMFm Policy Framework, Implementation and Business Plan set out in the Board's decision at the Seventeenth Board Meeting (GF/B17/DP16).

The committee shall report directly to the Board and shall consult with other committees as appropriate in developing its recommendations and advice to the Board.

Source: GFATM. Report of Affordable Medicines Facility — Malaria Ad Hoc Committee. The Global Fund Nineteenth Board Meeting GF/B19/7, Geneva, Switzerland, May 5–6, 2009 10/10.

4.7. Challenges in the Macroenvironment

On February 4, 2011, the Executive Directors of the GFATM and the RBM Partnership coconvened a forum in Geneva for the "AMFm Founders" to examine progress and share perspectives on challenges that needed collective attention. The group included those who, in 2007, invited the GFATM to consider hosting and managing AMFm Phase 1, whose implementation started in mid-2010. The convenors aimed to: (a) share with participants an update on progress and challenges; (b) seek their perspectives and guidance on how to judge the success of AMFm

Phase 1, which was then scheduled to last from mid-2010 to mid-2012; and (c) seek their perspectives on potential scenarios for going global with the AMFm, in the event that Phase 1 succeeded. The following institutions were represented: African Leaders Malaria Alliance (ALMA), Bill & Melinda Gates Foundation, CHAI, Ghana Health Services, Global Fund Secretariat, UNICEF, UNITAID, Government of the United Kingdom (DFID), RBM Secretariat, WHO, and the World Bank. The Office of the UN Secretary General's Envoy for Malaria sent regrets and comments.

Their discussions included the following:

- The AMFm had amplified several preexisting issues. Addressing them was beyond the agreed scope of the AMFm, or the GFATM, or any single institution alone. It was important to clarify the responsibilities of various institutions.
- Africa-based manufacturers: The African Leaders Malaria Alliance and the RBM Partnership were leading an exercise to find options for increasing the number of Africa-based manufactures with WHO-prequalified products. The scope of the coalition working on this issue would be increased, and the products needed to include not only ACTs but also Rapid Diagnostic Tests (RDTs). Active engagement of Africa-based manufacturers was also good for sustainability.
- Price competitiveness: Even if such manufacturers gained prequalification, they might not be price competitive in the short run. Should the GFATM consider domestic price preference for prequalified products from Africa-based manufacturers?
- Diagnostics: WHO updated its guidelines regarding diagnostics after the GFATM Board had approved AMFm Phase 1. In mid-2010, the GFATM and WHO coconvened an expert consultation on the economics and financing of universal access to diagnostics for malaria. The meeting reaffirmed the need for universal access to diagnostics and also highlighted the complexities of the challenge, particularly in the private sector, which accounts for a significant part of presumptive treatment. Resolving these issues was beyond the AMFm alone, but the AMFm business model might contribute to a faster and more widespread use of RDTs. Although the use of RDTs was outside the immediate proof of concept of the AMFm, the AMFm served as a

driver and identifier of pathways for expanding the use of RDTs. If the AMFm business model proved effective for ACTs, it could pave the way for an expansion of scope that would include RDTs.

- Changes in the local regulatory framework: Regulations and enforcement capacities varied across countries. They affected the potential reach of ACTs even when there were subsidized products.
- Taxes and tariffs: The elimination of taxes and tariffs would help to reduce the retail price to users. There had been recent progress on these in Ghana and Nigeria, but much remained to be done in most places.

4.8. Oxfam versus the Poor

According to its self-description on the Oxfam website,

> "Oxfam International was formed in 1995 by a group of independent non-governmental organizations. They joined together as a confederation to maximize efficiency and achieve greater impact to reduce global poverty and injustice. The name "Oxfam" comes from the Oxford Committee for Famine Relief, founded in Britain in 1942."[31]

One might take at face value the assertion of commitment to reducing global poverty and injustice. However, in the case of the AMFm, Oxfam was a liability to the cause of reducing poverty, an enabler of inefficiency, and a barrier to disciplined learning.

In public and within the AMFm Ad Hoc Committee of the Global Fund Board, Oxfam's contributions to discourse were devoid of intellectual rigor. If the propensity for damage were limited to buffoonery, it might not have mattered much in the bigger picture. But their aversion to thoughtful engagement based on scientific evidence was multiplied by the vehemence of their ideological convictions that the public sector alone must do everything in the treatment of malaria, and by their implicit belief that they alone knew what was good for people in the lower income and wealth quintiles of malaria-endemic countries. So extreme was Oxfam's evidence-free conviction that, in a global contest of irrational fanaticism, they would have won the gold medal.

But there was a nefarious method to Oxfam's madness. Many NGOs from the Global North do serious work and contribute much to health discourse and services in some of the hardest-to-reach places in the Global South. Those NGOs are thoughtful, diligent, compassionate, and open to learning alongside institutions and persons whose starting perspectives might lie outside the traditional comfort zones of the NGOs. They recognize that just as they might be right on any particular issue, they might be wrong. Unfortunately, global health is rife with the self-conferred presumption of omniscience and a self-mounted halo of sainthood by a subset of NGOs from the Global North, of which Oxfam was the poster child. Since neither their institutional legitimacy nor funding derives from any electoral mandate, direct or otherwise, from the populations of the Global South, they are not accountable to that population. NGOs in this select category share two key traits. First, they are happy only when they are miserable. Second, they supposedly do not want global institutions to dictate policies to countries of the Global South, but they relentlessly seek to influence, bully, or harass global institutions into pushing onto the Global South the preferences of those NGOs. It is a classic case of claiming unearned authority without accountability.

Oxfam's ignorance was on full display in its February 2009 report entitled "Blind optimism: Challenging the myths about private health care in poor countries." The report provided no credible comparative analysis of public and private means to expand health care. But a lack of substance did not prevent Oxfam from decreeing its manifesto:[32]

> *"Governments and rich country donors must strengthen state capacities to regulate and focus on the rapid expansion of free publicly provided health care, a proven way to save millions of lives worldwide."*

If anything had been proven in LICs and LMICs, especially in the treatment of malaria, it was that the public sector *alone* was incapable of delivering basic health services to the population on a large scale. Yet, in a rhetorical sleight of hand, Oxfam zealously advocated for the continuation of those failed policies. So shoddy was the Oxfam report that it received a commentary entitled "Oxfam — This is Not How To Help the Poor,"[33] which concluded as follows:

"This Oxfam report aims for a leap backward — to the days when all efforts to help the poor were unthinkingly focused on the public providers that we like, and feel comfortable with. We know now that the poor go where they want to go, and they will persist in doing so. The choice we face is, do we acknowledge this and overcome our discomfort with these untrained people who make their living by selling their services and products or do we not? Clearly, for Oxfam, the answer is no. And, with this report, they would answer not only for their own efforts, but for everyone in the global community. If we listen, we are giving in to wishful thinking, and at the expense of finding ways to improve the lives of the poor."

Thus, an NGO with Oxfamian inclinations could access and seek to hold sway over public policy. That was made the more egregious by the fact that their representation and professional preparations were often mediocre compared to those of bona fide representatives of governments and other institutions from the Global South who wanted to empirically explore options to improve access to affordable medicines in their own countries. In hindsight, Oxfam's preening becomes tragicomical when juxtaposed against the dehumanizing conduct of some of its staff who engaged in sexual exploitation of vulnerable people in some of the countries that Oxfam claims to serve. It reportedly took the threat of de-funding by the UK-DFID for Oxfam to come clean:[34–36]

"Mordaunt said Oxfam had told her department "categorically no" when it had asked if any aid beneficiaries had been involved in or affected by the misconduct. Asked if that was a lie, Mordaunt said: "Well, quite."

Oxfam said it now had a dedicated safeguarding team, a confidential whistleblowing hotline and safeguarding contact point within countries, and a code of conduct that stipulated: "I will also not exchange money, offers of employment, employment, goods or services for sex or sexual favors.""

To safeguard the Global South from the intellectual equivalent of sexual exploitation, Oxfam should implement a code of conduct that stipulates:

"We will neither pontificate outside our circle of competence nor presume that Oxfam knows best in matters of health in the Global South."

Oxfam thus came to the AMFm with a certitude that was untroubled by careful reflection and facts. Proceeding with a creed that it was their way or the highway, they would harangue and harass, and they were permanently angry. They would tie up deliberations of the AMFm Ad Hoc Committee and waste inordinate amounts of the time of the AMFm team over minutiae.

Marketing was a central element of the private sector dimension of AMFm Phase 1. Accordingly, and following careful consultations with individuals and parties with deep subject matter expertise, the AMFm team recommended the adoption of a logo to distinguish AMFm co-paid ACTs from others. It was a simple and thoughtful case of branding a product to distinguish it from others and to convey a promise to the buyer: you are buying a quality product that is subsidized by the AMFm and good for your health. It was as basic as the swoosh on a Nike shoe. This also made sense in light of a clamor by Oxfam and the US-PMI that AMFm must demonstrate its market performance relative to other approaches. Yet, Oxfam vehemently objected to the use of an AMFm-specific logo as a branding tool.[37] This, among many other occasions, demonstrated Oxfam's gleeful aversion to reason and their substitution of drama for diligence.

One of the most dishonest ploys of Oxfam, which it shared with one other member of the AMFm Ad Hoc Committee, was an aversion to the basic concept of comparing alternative approaches on similar criteria and timelines as a basis for informing policy. In this particular feature, Oxfam had kindred spirits in the US-PMI.

4.9. US-PMI: *We Are the Law*

USAID, which had commissioned the initial work led by Arrow, was remarkably incurious about empirically testing the IOM's recommendations published in *Saving Lives, Buying Time*. It provided no coherent rationale for that position; surely nothing as rigorous and thorough as *Saving Lives, Buying Time*. USAID was unhappy and vengeful because

Arrow and others told it what it needed to know instead of what it preferred to hear. But if USAID had wanted a sycophantic report in the first instance, it should not have asked the IOM Committee that included some of the best informed and independent thinkers across malariology, public health, and economics. More importantly, during implementation of AMFm Phase 1, the US-PMI's disposition to the AMFm was a combination of vicious hostility and detestation to undermine the innovation. They tried early and often to hobble the AMFm. They contributed nothing to the AMFm co-payment fund but sought to limit how many ACTs the AMFm could pay for. The implication was stunning: *US-PMI, which insisted that the AMFm must prove perfection, asked that the AMFm should run at suboptimal capacity while proving that perfection.* This was just one example of US-PMI's disingenuity. Having declared the AMFm unworthy before it was launched, they devoted their enormous resources to crusading against it.

Some of the scorched-earth strategy deployed by US-PMI played out through the AMFm Ad Hoc Committee of the GFATM Board, which oversaw the GFATM Secretariat's implementation of the AMFm. Some publicly available records of the GFATM Board and the AMFm Ad Hoc Committee, even in their sanitized language of a bureaucracy that was calibrated to avoid the ire of the GFATM's largest donor, reveal to discerning observers what was transpiring behind the scenes. The following is an excerpt from a report on the deliberations of the AMFm Ad Hoc Committee (AHC) at its meeting and conference calls in September and October 2009. It refers to progress in preparations for the launch of AMFm Phase 1 and the Committee's recommendations to the GFATM Board's 20th Meeting, held in Addis Ababa (report GF/B20/7 of November 2009):

"AMFm Ad Hoc Committee membership.

2.17. In advance of the Committee's meeting of 1–2 October 2009, the US constituency advised the Committee Chair, Board Chair and Vice-Chair, and the Secretariat on 25 September that it was resigning its membership of the AMFm Ad Hoc Committee with immediate effect, in order to take up a position on the Ad Hoc Market Dynamics Committee (MDC). The Committee Chair accepted the US constituency's resignation. The US representative therefore did not participate in the Committee meeting of 1–2 October and its teleconference of 12 October; however, the Committee took account of the US constituency's position on a variety of issues, as formally communicated in their resignation letter. Members of the AMFm Ad Hoc Committee appreciate the contributions of the US representative to issues discussed on AMFm at the Committee level. The AMFm Ad Hoc Committee also understands that the rule that limits membership by constituencies to two committees does not apply to the AMFm and MDC Ad Hoc Committees. (The two-committee limit was specifically excluded by the Board when the AMFm and MDC committees were established). Therefore, members of the AMFm Ad Hoc Committee strongly encourage the US to reconsider its decision so that its representative can continue to contribute as a member of the AMFm Ad Hoc Committee."

US-PMI haughtily presumed that its business model was above all others. But it would neither subject its business model to anything close to the methodical evaluation of the AMFm nor agree to comparative analysis using similar criteria over a similar period of implementation. US-PMI was never interested in seeing the methodical and rigorous evaluation of AMFm Phase 1 if that meant any chance that the AMFm might succeed and proceed beyond Phase 1. *It was not a matter of playing by shared laws: US-PMI was the law!* They would, of course, spew platitudes about respect for scientific evidence, but that was just a hollow ritual. They would not participate in forums aimed at discussing in neutral ways the construct, progress, and challenges facing the AMFm. Some staff of contractors to US-PMI, speaking on condition of anonymity for fear of retaliation and losing their contracts, informed the AMFm team that they were instructed by US-PMI not to participate in certain consultations about or involving the AMFm. Some country officials, also speaking on condition of anonymity for fear of having US-PMI abruptly terminate funding for programs in their countries, informed the AMFm team that US-PMI warned them not to participate in AMFm Phase 1. The independent evaluation of US-PMI included the following:"[38]

"Several people from the Global Fund and the RBM partnership were critical of PMI's position on the Affordable Medicines Facility-malaria (AMFm). They believe that PMI asks for a higher level of proof than other initiatives and seems antagonistic to AMFm. The perception expressed was that PMI/USAID works against AMFm approval by Global Fund Board and tends to undermine the facility."

"PMI was not seen as a good partner in one specific area. PMI leadership and selected technical personnel may have their reservations about AMFm, but the evaluation team heard from multiple sources that the perception of an openly antagonistic manner in which PMI voices its concerns is unjustified and potentially inappropriate."

Those were under-statements. In a destructive campaign, US-PMI essentially bullied or sought to bully any entity that did not serve its purpose. It found willing collaborators within parts of the GFATM while Kazatchkine — who was exemplary in his commitment to testing the AMFm as a concept — was still Executive Director of the GFATM, and it had free rein after Kazatchkine left the GFATM in March 2012.[39]

In hindsight, even though these events took place while the honorable Barack Obama was President of the United States, the methods employed by US-PMI in matters of the AMFm were strikingly similar to what the world later came to see during the presidency of Donald Trump. Regarding the AMFm, US-PMI practiced Trumpism well before Trump took center stage: the toxic hostility; the celebration of *alternative facts*; the emasculation of the befuddled leadership of that period's Global Malaria Program of WHO; the spurious arguments; the specious pronouncements instead of a respect for evidence from the independent evaluation;[40] and the bullying of the GFATM (Secretariat, AMFm Ad Hoc Committee, and the Board). That said, one must give US-PMI credit where it is due; they never asked anyone to drink bleach as a cure for malaria. Not in public, at least.

4.10. Preemptively Undermining an Independent Evaluation

"Their hypocrisy is both a tribute to the growing rationality of man and a proof of the ease with which rational demands may be circumvented."

—Reinhold Niebuhr[e]

The GFATM Board had an epistemological problem when it came to its oversight and leadership regarding the independent evaluation of AMFm Phase 1: contrary to the zeal for fundraising and traditional grant-making, there was *de facto* no Board commitment to methodical learning and no willingness to let the evidence lead where it might. The hegemonic machination of the wealthiest Board constituency and the ideology of the loudest Board constituency mattered more than conclusions based on scientific rigor. That debacle was years in the making.

4.10.1 The epistemological problem

The GFATM commissioned a study to estimate benchmarks of success of AMFm Phase 1, with a view to enabling an objective decision on the findings of an independent evaluation.[41,42] A benchmark is only as good as the willingness of the decider to use it and let the evidence lead where it might. The GFATM Board was not enthusiastic about making evidence-based decisions on the AMFm if doing so would displease its wealthiest Board member.

A key challenge was how to match the duration of in-country implementation of the AMFm with an AMFm evaluation design that would be rigorous and appropriate for a proof of concept. The goal-post kept shifting but the rationale was never based on logic. In fact, it was internally incoherent in light of the stark observation from the GFATM's own Five-Year Evaluation Report, and optimized not for learning but to please the most powerful and wealthiest constituency of the GFATM Board. At its

---

[e]Niebuhr R. 1932. *Moral Man and Immoral Society. A Study in Ethics and Politics.* Louisville: Westminster John Knox Press. p. 95.

17th meeting (April 2008), the Global Fund Board decided as follows (Annex 1 to Decision Point GF/B17/DP8):[43]

> *"Expansion from the initial phase to a full roll out in all eligible countries will occur within a year of launch unless clear failures ("red flags") in the AMFm design are observed."*

Two constituencies of the GFATM Board sought to pre-fix the evaluation such that it would be virtually impossible for the AMFm to be judged a success. The AMFm Ad Hoc Committee (AHC)'s report to the 20th GFATM Board meeting of November 2009 included the following text (paragraph 4.4. of the report):[37]

> *"The AHC is aware that a 12 month implementation timeline presents issues regarding the parameters of the evaluation given the difficulty of measuring success in 12 months. In particular, since the Seventeenth Board meeting, some constituencies have stated that AMFm Phase 1 must provide definitive proof of attributable increases in ACT use among the poorest and most remote populations. The majority of AHC members acknowledge that this is not a realistic expectation within 12 months in the context of many implementing countries. AMFm is a new business model without direct precedent in global health. ACTs are no longer new technologies, but co-paid ACTs will be new. In the Final Report of the Global Fund Five-Year Evaluation: Study Area 3, it was noted that "The findings related to ACTs are the most perplexing and worrisome of the four primary malaria interventions because they show the least improvement." A key lesson from the Five-year Evaluation relates to the timeline for measurable changes that can be attributed to a new intervention or business model: "Most importantly, five years is an extraordinarily limited amount of time over which to measure global level outcomes and impact, especially in a new program with a new model. Investments of both new resources and new approaches require time to take root and bear fruit".[44]*
>
> *The AHC will work to define reasonable parameters for success or otherwise of AMFm Phase 1, based on the Monitoring and Evaluation Technical Framework and the timeline for implementation. The Developed Country NGOs constituency expressed a concern that, in*

measuring the use of ACTs, the Monitoring and Evaluation Technical framework would measure not only malaria specific fevers but fevers due to other causes. The Developed Country NGOs constituency also wished to have it noted that in their opinion, impact of AMFm on use of co-paid ACTs among the poorest and remote populations must form the basis for a "red flag" regardless of the evaluation period, and they would not compromise on this."

The GFATM Board then made the following decision at its 20th meeting (November 2009): (Decision Point GF/B20/DP24):[45]

"The Board refers to its earlier decisions regarding the Affordable Medicine Facility — malaria ("AMFm") and clarifies its intent that the Global Fund will only expand from Phase 1 (the pilot phase) of AMFm to a global scale-up on the basis of evidence gathered during the pilot phase that the initiative is likely to achieve its four stated objectives: (i) increased ACT affordability, (ii) increased ACT availability, (iii) increased ACT use, including among vulnerable groups, and (iv) "crowding out" oral artemisinin monotherapies, chloroquine and sulfadoxine-pyrimethamine by gaining market share. The Board further clarifies that it will consider evidence that the AMFm will achieve these four objectives more cost-effectively than other financing models that aim to achieve similar objectives solely or principally through the expansion of public sector services (i.e., public health facilities and community health workers only)."

For those opposed to the AMFm and averse to evidence, the preemptive fix was in at the decision level. That fix was regardless of the independence of the evaluation, which was an intellectually honest exercise and a rare undertaking in global health in scale and rigor. The ploy was clear: since the independent evaluation itself could not be corrupted, the feasible approach to killing the AMFm was to bully the deciders (i.e., the GFATM Board and its AMFm Ad Hoc Committee) and cow them into making wishy-washy decisions devoid of intellectual rigor. It was the development equivalent of a group preparing to storm the United States Capitol to overturn the result of a presidential election by bullying the constitutionally mandated electoral college because that group did not like the hard data coming from the election.

By the end of the first quarter of 2012, AMFm Phase 1 implementation was well underway and the firms contracted by the GFATM for the independent evaluation had started their work. We had gone where nobody ever had at the frontiers of private–public innovation for financing and delivering malaria medicines. An assignment that I had expected to last 2 years had been extended into a little over three years because it took much longer than anticipated to get the AMFm experiment fully underway. It was time to move on. In May 2012, I left the Global Fund in Geneva and returned to the World Bank in Washington DC. Emmanuel Yuniwo Nfor was my successor at the AMFm.

4.11. The Independent Evaluation

The GFATM commissioned an independent evaluation of the AMFm. The evaluation, projected to cost at least US$10 million, was intended to serve as the basis on which the GFATM Board would decide the future of the AMFm. Following a competitive selection process, the GFATM contracted ICF International and the London School of Hygiene and Tropical Medicine (LSHTM) to conduct the Independent Evaluation. The following are excerpts from the full report of the independent evaluation, dated September 28, 2012:[46]

> "*Achievement of success benchmarks* — *Figure 1 (in the report) provides an overview of the performance of each pilot against the AMFm success benchmarks. Of the 8 pilots, success benchmarks were clearly met in 5 pilots for availability, 5 pilots for QAACT price relative to the most popular antimalarial that is not a QAACT, and 4 pilots for QAACT market share (all shaded green). It is also possible that benchmarks were met in one additional pilot for availability and price, and in 3 additional pilots for market share, although the evidence is not as strong (shaded amber). The success benchmarks related to artemisinin monotherapy (AMT) price and market share were met in all pilots with sufficient AMTs in the market to make these benchmarks relevant.*"
>
> "*AMFm and the private for-profit sector* — *AMFm has been a "game changer" in the private for-profit sector for all pilots except Niger and Madagascar, with a dramatic impact on the antimalarial market, through large increases in QAACT availability, decreases in*

QAACT prices, and increases in QAACT market share. These changes were substantial and achieved in only a few months, demonstrating the power of tapping into the distributional capacity of the private sector. The changes are very likely to be largely attributable to AMFm. The private for-profit sector response was similar in rural and urban areas, in some cases reducing or closing a rural-urban gap in availability and market share. There was considerable penetration of copaid QAACTs even in remote areas in Ghana and Kenya, where this was evaluated."

*"**Effect of duration of implementation** — Longer duration of implementation appears to be positively correlated with performance, if the combined presence of copaid ACTs and the operation of a large-scale sustained IEC/BCC campaign is considered a proxy for full AMFm implementation. With the exception of Zanzibar, pilots with earlier start dates achieved more success benchmarks. No large-scale sustained IEC/ BCC campaign was in place by the end of 2011 in Madagascar, Niger or Uganda, and these pilots achieved fewer benchmarks. However, it is possible that delayed start dates reflect weaker implementation capacity in general, and therefore one should be cautious in attributing performance to duration of implementation alone.*

The characterization of the AMFm as a game changer was no surprise to those who had been observing the implementation of the AMFm. It was a matter of fact. By contrast, the traditional business model of the GFATM was sclerotic, slow, and prone to repetitive glitches. If the AMFm innovation was a robust Ferrari, the traditional GFATM business model for malaria medicines was a lumbering — and sickly — snail.

A short version of findings from the independent evaluation was published in *The Lancet* in October 2012.[47] As of the time of the independent evaluation, funding had amounted to US$336 million for ACT co-payments (from Canada, the United Kingdom, UNITAID, and the Bill and Melinda Gates Foundation), and US$127 million for supporting interventions (from the GFATM). From August 2010 to December 2011, the AMFm had financed 155.8 million doses of quality-assured ACTs, which had been delivered to the participating countries.

The independent evaluation found that "In all pilots except Niger and Madagascar, there were large increases in QAACT availability (25.8–51.9 percentage points), and market share (15.9–40.3 percentage points), driven mainly by changes in the private for-profit sector. Large falls in median price for QAACTs per adult equivalent dose were seen in the private for-profit sector in six pilots, ranging from US$1.28 to US$4.82. The market share of oral artemisinin monotherapies decreased in Nigeria and Zanzibar, the two pilots where it was more than 5% at baseline." It further noted that:

> *"Subsidies combined with supporting interventions can be effective in rapidly improving availability, price, and market share of QAACTs, particularly in the private for-profit sector."*

When judged by preestablished benchmarks[48,49] and the independent evaluation, the AMFm was a success. The preestablished benchmarks provided a basis for answering the "compared to what?" question. As of November 2012, when the GFATM Board decided on the future of the AMFm, there was no other published independent evaluation, of similar rigor and scale, of approaches to the improvement of access to malaria medicines.

4.12. Bullying the Global Fund Board

> *"Facts are stubborn things; and whatever may be our wishes, our inclinations, or the dictates of our passions, they cannot alter the state of facts and evidence…"*

—John Adams

4.12.1 Unremitting opposition despite the evidence

Despite the prior work on benchmarks and evidence from the independent evaluation, the decision of the GFATM on the future of the AMFm took place in an atmosphere that was defined and dominated by US-PMI's obdurate and vehement crusade against the AMFm. Debates about the AMFm included and/or covered originators of the study that underpinned the AMFm, longstanding opponents of the AMFm, financiers of alternative and hitherto unsuccessful approaches to improve effective access to ACTs for malaria (to which the successful AMFm was therefore a competitor), observers who strongly preferred government-run approaches to the financing, distribution, and prescription of malaria medicines, independent think tanks, academics, and managers of malaria control programs in African countries. Some raised questions about whether or not the decision was made on the merit of the case, or on other considerations, and asked whether the decision was a way to kill a successful but politically inconvenient innovation.[50–57]

US-PMI had the track record of hostility, the motive — to destroy the AMFm, the means — via the leverage that the United States had over the GFATM, and the opportunity — a GFATM Board decision — to kill the AMFm:

> *"Although a pilot, AMFm was introduced as a total country program in seven countries that represent a quarter of the world's malaria cases and has transformed access to effective antimalarials. However, the value of AMFm was challenged by the US President's Malaria Initiative (PMI) well before it was ever put in place. According to an independent assessment of PMI, key experts noted that "PMI/USAID works against AMFm approval by the Global Fund Board and tends to undermine the facility". With the world's largest global health funder expressing unremitting opposition, even after the positive independent evaluation, the program's future is uncertain. PMI has yet to suggest an alternative that would come close to the access afforded by AMFm in the private sector."[56]*

African Malaria Control Program managers called for a decision based on the merit of the case:[53]

> *"AMFm has proven itself and should be expanded to include more countries and adapted as needed to the changing malaria landscape and country specific context. This may mean finding ways of encouraging the use of RDTs, for instance. But the basic architecture of the AMFm subsidy and price negotiations should continue and expand. The evidence supports AMFm and the cost is not prohibitive for what it delivers. The $300 million spent on the pilot is a mere fraction of the $30 billion or so of the health development aid spent around the world each year. The credibility of the international community in Africa is at stake. AMFm should be a global priority, not merely an interesting footnote of malaria control history."*

4.13. Meet the American Development Industrial Complex

If the AMFm were expanded, its proven effectiveness in using the supply chains of domestic private sector firms would become an existential threat to the entrenched business model of USAID and US-PMI, which funded large American contractors to run supply chains and deliver medicines in many LICs and LMICs. The entrenched system stood to lose — and possibly collapse — if the innovative business model of the AMFm became the standard for procuring malaria medicines and other commodities, and for working through locally-owned and locally-managed supply chains (instead of through American contractors). The AMFm had shown that *the natives*, who had been framed as uncomfortable with shoes and unable to tell the time of day with wristwatches, could run their own affairs. Its continuation had troubling implications for the *status quo*.

The reader is encouraged to study an insightful article on a concurrent upheaval, which was published in July 2012. In that article, John Norris unpacked efforts by USAID Administrator Rajiv Shah in a "high-stakes battle to make US foreign aid programs less dependent on American for-profit contractors." That was in the context of a fact that might be startling to people who were not paying attention to the *systemic* mess of the business models of USAID and US-PMI: in 2011 the 10 largest USAID contractors received more than US\$3.19 billion. Against that entrenched system, Shah was pushing to route funds directly to institutions in the Global South, including governments, entrepreneurs, educational institutions, and NGOs. The article included a searing indictment of the *status quo*:[58]

> *"Given the degree to which USAID works with contractors, some of Shah's language has been delightfully undiplomatic. In a 2011 speech, he drew parallels between the agency's reliance on for-profit firms and Eisenhower's warnings about the emergence of a military-industrial complex. Saying that USAID was "no longer satisfied with writing big checks to big contractors and calling it development," Shah argued that development firms were more interested in keeping themselves in business than seeing countries graduate from the need for aid. "There is always another high-priced consultant that must take another flight to attend another conference or lead another training," he complained."*

The American contractors' reaction to Shah's initiative was swift and ferocious.[59] Almost a decade later, the business model of USAID and US-PMI remains essentially unchanged.

4.14. Choosing Mediocrity: GFATM Board Kills the AMFm

Based on its objectives, prespecified success benchmarks, and the independent evaluation, the AMFm succeeded as a proof of concept on a scale rarely seen in global health, and within an extraordinarily short period. It demonstrated the effectiveness of a combination of price negotiations, factory-gate subsidy, and the use of domestic private sector importers, domestic private sector supply chains and outlets, to dramatically improve affordability, availability, and access to life-saving malaria medicines.

The traditional business model clearly hadn't worked for malaria medicines even after its first five years, as noted in the Five-Year Evaluation of the GFATM. The AMFm, after just one year of effective implementation, had performed far better than any known alternative for the specified purposes. But the facts from the independent evaluation and the calls for evidence-based decision, including from African program leaders, stood no chance against hegemonic bullying of the GFATM Board by its largest financier. In the period leading up to the GFATM Board meeting, the GFATM Secretariat and Board, being financially beholden to the United States, faced the development equivalent of a Faustian bargain. The GFATM could either grovel to its largest financier or stand with integrity on findings from the independent evaluation. The need to secure continued funding for the GFATM's traditional business model — of grants for AIDS, TB, and malaria programs — was being addressed amidst fears of angering the United States delegation to the GFATM Board and US-PMI. In October 2012, the GFATM Secretariat was concerned about securing assurances from the United States constituency that all domestic United States legislative restrictions had been addressed. Given Kazatchkine's departure several months earlier, there was no longer the executive leadership with the combination of intellectual credibility, strategic vision, and fortitude to stand up for using science to inform the Board's decision.

In November 2012, the GFATM Board decided to kill the AMFm. In a piece of disingenuous wordsmithing, it decided to "modify the existing AMFm business line by integrating the lessons learned from the operations and resourcing of Phase 1 of the AMFm into Global Fund grant management and financial processes," and noted that "the integration of a co-payment system into Global Fund grant management and financial processes will mean that, following a responsible Transition, co-payments for anti-malarial drugs will no longer be available through a separate funding mechanism hosted by the Global Fund."[60]

The GFATM Board's decision to "integrate" the AMFm into the traditional business model was a political sleight of hand to suffocate an innovation that its largest and dominant financier wanted dead. Faced with a choice between progress based on innovation and transparent learning on the one hand, and the familiar mediocrity of its traditional approach on the other hand, the GFATM Board chose the latter:[50]

> "On Nov 15, the Board of the Global Fund to Fight AIDS, Tuberculosis and Malaria announced its verdict on the question of whether to "expand, accelerate, terminate or suspend"[61] the Affordable Medicines Facility — malaria (AMFm): AMFm would be "integrated" into the existing grant proposal process. This strategy, at face value, is no different from what the Fund was doing before AMFm. (Countries were able to engage in national-level subsidies, but did not.) The Fund's decision to return to "business as usual" is difficult to understand.
>
> The Global Fund and other AMFm financiers (the UK Government, Gates Foundation, and UNITAID) deserve praise for their audacity to try AMFm at scale, and to commit resources for evaluation. AMFm is the Fund's only multicountry experiment, and the evaluation (Dec 1, p 1916)[62] is the Fund's only deliberate attempt at rigorous, albeit imperfect, impact assessment.
>
> Yet the ultimate role played by the evaluation's evidence is unclear. Many questions remain unanswered, including how lessons from the experiment will be incorporated into the grant proposal process, or what incentives countries will have to opt into a subsidy. Also unknown is how countries will cope with this sudden policy shift.

This one-off experiment holds crucial implications for the general role of experiments in policy making by donors and development organisations. How can the global health community thoughtfully permit, or enable, experimentation and learning? Experimentation, innovation, and learning are technically difficult, resource-intensive, and are often threatening to long-held ideas and interests and to long-term planning. Isolated trials and rhetoric are not enough. Done well, and with appropriate country participation, this process holds tremendous promise."

There is no publicly available record of rigorously scientific methods, if any, adopted by proceedings of the Committee that informed the November 2012 GFATM Board decision, including its peer-reviewed analyses, if any, of the cost-effectiveness and efficiency of the AMFm compared to the traditional business model into which it was being integrated. It is important to recall that before the AMFm, the 5-year evaluation of the Global Fund reported the following on the traditional business model:

"The findings related to ACTs are the most perplexing and worrisome of the four primary malaria interventions because they show the least improvement."[44]

That under-performing traditional business model was the one into which the AMFm would now be integrated,[63] much like a surgeon choosing to graft fresh tissue onto necrotic tissue. The GFATM Board had committed the modern equivalent of denying that the earth moved around the sun.

4.15. *Eppur si muove!*[f]

The AMFm worked. It was also too successful to survive in an ecosystem that thrived on mediocrity and rent seeking. Its case illustrates some of the

---

[f]"And yet it moves." This phrase has been attributed to Galileo Galilei, with reference to the Catholic Church's doctrine that the earth stood still and was the center of the universe. Galileo held that the Church's model was wrong. *Source:* Livio M. 2020. Did Galileo truly say, 'and yet it moves'? A modern detective story. *Scientific American.* https://

promise of disruptive innovation and the dysfunctional dynamics of decision-making in DAH. This, in turn, raises unanswered questions about the extent to which independent evidence informs or drives important decisions, and the extent to which political considerations trump such evidence, even when the evidence is clear and compelling. It also raises questions about the ultimate beneficiaries of such development assistance,[58,64,65] whether and how domestic dysfunctions within donor countries affect the manner in which they pursue bilateral development assistance,[66] and what reforms might be useful to ensure greater transparency of decision-making. This is especially important, as the AMFm's then-new architecture of development assistance demonstrated that local private sector supply chains were very effective, hence there was no need to continue channeling development assistance largely or exclusively through dysfunctional government medical stores and supply chains, and there was no need for traditional approaches to bilateral development assistance in which external contractors established and managed separate supply chain projects within recipient countries.

This case also raises a question about whether the decision process would have been transparent and more robust had the hosting and management of AMFm Phase 1 been separated from the right and duty to decide whether or not the innovation would be expanded, and which institution or group of institutions would be eligible to host and manage it in a second phase. A global version of the National Institute for Health and Care Excellence (NICE),[67] acting with a combination of intellectual integrity, independence from financiers of DAH, and political insulation from lobbyists at any part of the private-public ideological spectrum, might improve the transparency and credibility of such decisions in the context of global health and DAH.

Elements of the AMFm approach — price negotiations, supra-national subsidies, and use of in-country private sector supply chains, can be used for other health technologies, including diagnostics and treatments for acute respiratory tract infections, diarrheal diseases, and potentially for selected chronic, non-communicable diseases, especially in situations

---

blogs.scientificamerican.com/observations/did-galileo-truly-say-and-yet-it-moves-a-modern-detective-story/. Accessed on June 8, 2021.

where price is a barrier to access, and public-sector dominated supply chains are dysfunctional. Amidst the debacle of vaccine nationalism and lack of access to COVID-19 vaccines in most of the Global South, some researchers noted that the AMFm has already provided lessons for effective engagement with pharmaceutical companies.[68]

Almost a decade after the epic failure of its Board, the GFATM is yet to find a conceptually coherent and operationally robust way to engage with the commercial private sector in malaria medicines and diagnostics. An overhaul of USAID's and US-PMI's inferior and inefficient model of DAH[69] is long overdue. And the malaria parasite marches on.

References

[1] Frost LJ, Reich MR. 2009. *Access: How Do Good Health Technologies Get to Poor People in Poor Countries?* Cambridge: Harvard University Press.

[2] Adeyi O, Atun R. 2010. Universal access to malaria medicines: Innovation in financing and delivery. *The Lancet* , 376: 1869–1871. http://www.thelancet.com/pdfs/journals/lancet/PIIS0140-6736(10)61189-0.pdf. Accessed on January 19, 2021.

[3] Frost L, Reich MR, Pratt BA, Guyer AL. March 31, 2009. Process evaluation of the project on defining the architecture and management of a global subsidy for antimalarial drugs. http://siteresources.worldbank.org/INTMALARIA/Resources/AMFmProcessEvaluation.pdf. Accessed on January 19, 2021.

[4] Arrow KJ, Panosian C, Gelband H. Editors. 2004. Saving lives, buying time. In *Committee on the Economics of Antimalarial Drugs*. Board on Global Health. Institute of Medicines of the National Academies. The National Academies Press.

[5] WHO. 2006. *Guidelines for the Treatment of Malaria*. Geneva: World Health Organization.

[6] Frost LJ, Reich M. March 31, 2009. *Translating an Idea into a Policy: "Saving Lives and Buying Time" for Antimalarial Medicines.* Harvard School of Public Health Global Health Teaching Case. https://www.hsph.harvard.edu/michael-reich/teaching-cases-in-global-health/. Accessed on June 7, 2021.

[7] Bernstein PL. 1996. *Against the Gods. The Remarkable Story of Risk.* New York, NY: John Wiley & Sons Ltd. pp. 202–204.

[8] Laxminarayan R, Over M, Smith DL. 2006. Will a global subsidy of new antimalarials delay the emergence of resistance and save lives? *Health Affairs*, 25: 325–336.

[9] Roll Back Malaria Partnership. 2007. RBM Partnership Board gives the go ahead for the further development of an Affordable Medicines Facility — malaria (AMFm). https://www.malariaconsortium.org/news-centre/rbm_gives_go_ahead_for_development_of_amfm.htm. Accessed on January 22, 2021.

[10] The Nobel Prize. Linus Pauling. https://www.nobelprize.org/prizes/chemistry/1954/pauling/facts/. Accessed on January 21, 2021.

[11] Carpenter J. Nobel win for crystal discovery. https://www.bbc.com/news/science-environment-15181187. Accessed on January 21, 2021.

[12] Russell S. 2001. AIDS activists in uproar over official's remarks on Africa. https://www.sfgate.com/health/article/AIDS-activists-in-uproar-over-official-s-remarks-2911007.php.

[13] Committee on International Relations of the United States House of Representatives. June 7, 2001. *The United States' War on AIDS. Hearing before the 107th Congress*. First Session. pp. 107–117. http://commdocs.house.gov/committees/intlrel/hfa72978.000/hfa72978_0.HTM. Accessed on January 21, 2021.

[14] Kengor P, Doerner PC. 2007. *The Judge: William P. Clark, Ronald Reagan's Top Hand*. San Francisco: Ignatius Press. pp. 110–115.

[15] Kim S, Gerver SM, Fidler S. Ward H. August 24, 2014. Adherence to antiretroviral therapy in adolescents living with HIV systematic review and meta-analysis. *AIDS*, 28(13): 1945–1956. https://journals.lww.com/aidsonline/fulltext/2014/08240/adherence_to_antiretroviral_therapy_in_adolescents.12.aspx. Accessed on April 27, 2021.

[16] Nachega JB, Morroni C, Zuniga JM, Schechter M, Rockstroh J, Solomon S, Sherer R. 2012. HIV treatment adherence, patient health literacy, and health care provider–patient communication: Results from the 2010 AIDS Treatment for Life International Survey. JIAPAC. https://journals.sagepub.com/doi/10.1177/1545109712437244. Accessed on April 29, 2021.

[17] Nilsson J. 2015. How Tarzan's author did it all wrong and got it all right. https://www.saturdayeveningpost.com/2015/08/how-tarzans-author-did-it-all-wrong-and-got-it-right/. Accessed on January 22, 2025.

[18] Gambino L. 2019. Ronald Reagan called African UN delegates 'monkeys', recordings reveal. *The Guardian*. https://www.theguardian.com/us-news/2019/jul/31/ronald-reagan-racist-recordings-nixon. Accessed on January 25, 2021.

[19] Naftali T. 2019. Ronald Reagan's racist conversation with Richard Nixon. *The Atlantic*. https://www.theatlantic.com/ideas/archive/2019/07/ronald-reagans-racist-conversation-richard-nixon/595102/. Accessed on April 27, 2021.

[20] Herbert B. October 6, 2005. Impossible, ridiculous, repugnant. *New York Times*. https://www.nytimes.com/2005/10/06/opinion/impossible-ridiculous-repugnant.html. Accessed on April 21, 2021.

[21] National Public Radio. 2019. *Historian Discusses Recording of Reagan's Racist Comments Made to Nixon.* Washington DC. https://www.npr.org/2019/07/31/747041525/historian-discusses-recording-of-reagans-racists-comments-made-to-nixon. Accessed on April 27, 2021.

[22] United States Centers for Disease Control and Prevention. Media statement from CDC Director Rochelle P. Walensky, MD, MPH, on racism and health. CDC Online Newsroom. CDC. https://www.cdc.gov/media/releases/2021/s0408-racism-health.html. Accessed on April 21, 2021.

[23] Bhosle M, Balkrishnan R. 2007. Drug reimportation practices in the United States. *Therapeutics and Clinical Risk Management.* 3(1): 41–46. https://www.ncbi.nlm.nih.gov/pmc/articles/PMC1936287/#b13. Accessed on January 22, 2021.

[24] AMFm Task Force of the Roll Back Malaria Partnership. 2007. Affordable Medicines Facility–malaria (AMFm): technical design. November, 2007. https://web.archive.org/web/20110712095558/ http:/www.rbm.who.int/partnership/tf/globalsubsidy/AMFmTechProposal.pdf. Accessed on April 15, 2021.

[25] Sabot OJ, Mwita A, Cohen JM, Ipuge Y, Gordon M, Bishop D, Odhiambo M, Ward L, Goodman C. Piloting the global subsidy: The impact of subsidized artemisinin-based combination therapies distributed through private drug shops in rural Tanzania. https://journals.plos.org/plosone/article?id=10.1371/journal.pone.0006857. Accessed on January 22, 2021.

[26] GFATM, Report of the affordable medicines facility for malaria — Malaria Ad Hoc Committee (Decision GF/B18/7, 18th Board Meeting, New Delhi, India) November 7–8, 2008.

[27] The Global Fund. $225 million partnership to bring effective malaria drugs to all who need them. 2009. https://www.theglobalfund.org/en/news/2009-04-17-usd225-million-partnership-to-bring-effective-malaria-drugs-to-all-who-need-them/. Accessed on April 15, 2021.

[28] McNeil DG. 2009. Subsidy plan seeks to cut malaria drug cost. https://www.nytimes.com/2009/04/18/world/18malaria.html?_r=1&ref=world. Accessed on January 23, 2021.

[29] GFATM. May 5–6, 2009. Report of affordable medicines facility — malaria AD hoc committee. The Global Fund Nineteenth Board Meeting GF/B19/7. Geneva, Switzerland.

[30] Roll Back Malaria. 2011. Updated ACT prices under the Affordable Medicines Facility-malaria 1 March 2011 fact sheet. *Roll Back Malaria*, Geneva.

[31] Oxfam International. Our history. https://www.oxfam.org/en/our-history. Accessed on September 18, 2021.

[32] Oxfam. 2009. Blind Optimism: Challenging the myths about private health care in poor countries. Oxfam Briefing Paper. https://oxfamilibrary.openrepository.com/bitstream/handle/10546/114093/bp125-blind-optimism-010209-en.pdf;jsess

ionid=36E8A3EFCD55716503326C4FB3137B41?sequence=1. Accessed on October 16, 2021.

[33] Harding A. 2009. Oxfam — This is Not How To Help the Poor. https://www. cgdev.org/blog/oxfam-%E2%80%94-not-how-help-poor. Accessed on January 18, 2021.

[34] Elgot J. 2018. Oxfam told to show 'moral leadership' or lose government funds: Minister says charity must hand over all its information on use of prostitutes in Haiti. *The Guardian*. https://www.theguardian.com/world/2018/feb/11/oxfam-show-moral-leadership-lose-government-funds-prostitutes-haiti. Accessed on January 18, 2021.

[35] Timeline: Oxfam sexual exploitation scandal in Haiti, Oxfam | *The Guardian*. https://www.theguardian.com/world/2018/jun/15/timeline-oxfam-sexual-exploitation-scandal-in-haiti. Accessed on January 26, 2021.

[36] Charity Commission for England and Wales. 2019. Inquiry Report: Summary Findings and Conclusions. Oxfam. Registered charity number 202918. https://assets.publishing.service.gov.uk/government/uploads/system/uploads/attachment_data/file/807943/Inquiry_Report_summary_findings_and_conclusions_Oxfam.pdf. Accessed on October 27, 2021.

[37] GFATM. Report of the affordable medicines facility — malaria (AMFM) ad hoc committee (AHC). Twentieth Board Meeting Addis Ababa, Ethiopia, November 9–11, 2009. GF/B20/7 Decision. p. 22.

[38] External Evaluation of the President's Malaria Initiative. 2011. Final report. Report No. 11-01-545). Document submitted by The QED Group, LLC, with CAMRIS International and Social & Scientific Systems, Inc., to the United States Agency for International Development under USAID Contract No. GHS-I-00-05-00005-0. pp. 40–41. https://pdf.usaid.gov/pdf_docs/Pdact333.pdf. Accessed on July 27, 2021.

[39] Kazatchkine M. 2012. Reflections on the global fund. *An Open Letter from Michel Kazatchkine*. http://www.michelkazatchkine.com/?page___&paged=9. Accessed on January 26, 2021.

[40] U.S. President's Malaria Initiative. 2012. AMFm and PMI's commitment to global efforts to ensure prompt malaria diagnosis and treatment. https://www.pmi.gov/news/in-the-press/news-full-view/amfm-and-pmi-s-commitment-to-global-efforts-to-ensure-prompt-malaria-diagnosis-and-treatment. Accessed on January 23, 2021.

[41] Schäferhoff M, Yamey G. 2011. Estimating benchmarks of success in the affordable medicines facility — malaria (AMFm) phase 1. www.seekdevelopment.org/e2pi_estimating_benchmarks_in_amfm_report_en.pdf. Accessed August 20, 2016.

[42] Schäferhoff M, Yamey G, Montagu D. 2012. Piloting the affordable medicines facility-malaria: What will success look like? *Bulletin of the World Health*

Organization, 90:452–460. http://www.who.int/bulletin/volumes/90/6/11-091199/en/. Accessed on August 20, 2016.

[43] The global fund to fight AIDS, tuberculosis, and malaria. Seventeenth Board Meeting. Geneva. Annex 1 to Decision Point GF/B17/DP8: Principles for AMFm policy framework, implementation and business plan. https://www.theglobalfund.org/media/3685/bm17_boardmeeting_decisions_en.pdf. Accessed on June 7, 2021.

[44] The five-year evaluation of the global fund to fight AIDS, tuberculosis and malaria. synthesis of study areas 1, 2 and 3. March 2009. Page viii. https://www.theglobalfund.org/en/technical-evaluation-reference-group/evaluations/2009-five-year-evaluation/. Accessed on January 23, 2021.

[45] The global fund to fight AIDS, Tuberculosis, and Malaria. Twentieth Board Meeting Addis Ababa, Ethiopia 9–11 November 2009. https://www.theglobalfund.org/media/3204/bm20_boardmeeting_decisions_en.pdf. Accessed on June 7, 2021.

[46] AMFm Independent Evaluation Team. 2012. Independent evaluation of phase 1 of the Affordable Medicines Facility — malaria (AMFm), multi-country independent evaluation report: final report. Calverton, Maryland and London: ICF International and London School of Hygiene and Tropical Medicine. September 28, 2012. https://researchonline.lshtm.ac.uk/id/eprint/2869474/1/AMFm_2012IE Phase1FinalReportWithoutAppendices_Report_en%20%282%29.pdf. Accessed on February 23, 2021.

[47] Tougher S, the ACTwatch Group, Ye Y. *et al.* 2012. Effect of the Affordable Medicines Facility — malaria (AMFm) on the availability, price, and market share of quality-assured artemisinin-based combination therapies in seven countries: a before-and-after analysis of outlet survey data. *The Lancet,* 380(9857): 1916–1926. http://www.thelancet.com/journals/lancet/article/PIIS0140-6736(12)61732-2/fulltext. Accessed on February 23, 2021.

[48] Schäferhoff M, Yamey G. 2011. Estimating benchmarks of success in the Affordable Medicines Facility — malaria phase 1. San Francisco: Evidence-to-Policy Initiative. http://www.theglobalfund.org/documents/amfm/E2PI_EstimatingBenchmarksInAMFm_Report_en/. Accessed January 19, 2012.

[49] Yamey G, Schäferhoff M, Montagu D. 2012. Piloting the Affordable Medicines Facility — malaria: What will success look like? *Bulletin of the World Health Organization,* 90:452–460. https://www.who.int/bulletin/volumes/90/6/11-091199/en/. Accessed on January 26, 2021.

[50] Bump J, Fan VY, Lanthorn H, Yavuz E. 2012. In the Global Fund's court: Experimentation, evaluation, and the AMFm. *The Lancet* 380(9858). http://www.

thelancet.com/journals/lancet/article/PIIS0140-6736(12)62123-0/fulltext?rss=yes. Accessed on January 20, 2021.

[51] Fan V, Lanthorn H. 2012. The future of AMFm: Making sense from all the noise. http://www.cgdev.org/blog/future-amfm-making-sense-all-noise. Accessed on August 18, 2016.

[52] Fan V. 2012. The future of AMFm: Realpolitik and realistic options (Part II). http://www.cgdev.org/blog/future-amfm-realpolitik-and-realistic-options-part-ii. Accessed on August 18, 2016.

[53] Talisuna A, Adibaku S, Amojah C, Others. 2012. The affordable medicines facility-malaria—A success in peril. *Malaria Journal*, 11:370. https://malaria-journal.biomedcentral.com/articles/10.1186/1475-2875-11-370. Accessed on August 18, 2016.

[54] Fan V, Silverman R. 2012. A global health mystery: What's behind the US government opposition on AMFm?. http://www.cgdev.org/blog/global-health-mystery-what%E2%80%99s-behind-us-government-position-amfm. Accessed on August 18, 2016.

[55] Butler D. Malaria programme gets kiss of death from global fund. http://blogs.nature.com/news/2012/11/malaria-medicines-venture-gets-kiss-of-death-from-global-fund.html. Accessed on August 18, 2016.

[56] Arrow K, Danzon P, Gelband H. 2012. The Affordable Medicines Facility—malaria: Killing it slowly. *The Lancet*, 380(9857): 1889–1890. http://www.thelancet.com/journals/lancet/article/PIIS0140-6736%2812%2961843-1/fulltext Accessed on August 18, 2016.

[57] Arrow K. 2012, November 13. *Saving a Program that Saves Lives*. New York Times. http://www.nytimes.com/2012/11/14/opinion/saving-a-malaria-program-that-saves-lives.html?_r=0. Accessed on September 19, 2021.

[58] Norris J. 2012. Hired gun fight: Obama's aid chief takes on the development-industrial complex. *Foreign Policy*. http://foreignpolicy.com/2012/07/18/hired-gun-fight/. Accessed on August 20, 2016.

[59] Devex Editor. USAID contractors react to 'hired gun fight'. 2012. https://www.devex.com/news/usaidcontractors-react-to-hired-gun-fight-78752. Accessed on July 3, 2021.

[60] The Global Fund to Fight AIDS, Tuberculosis and Malaria. GF/B28/DP06. Integration of the Lessons from the Affordable Medicines Facility — malaria. Approved by the Board on 15 November 2012. http://www.theglobalfund.org/Knowledge/Decisions/GF/B28/DP06/. Accessed on August 18, 2016.

[61] Global Fund to fight AIDS tuberculosis and malaria. Report of the Affordable Medicines Facility — malaria Ad Hoc Committee. http://www.theglobalfund.org/

documents/board/18/BM18_07AMFmAdHocCommittee_Report_en/. In Bump, J., Fan VY, Lanthorn, H., Yavuz E. (Editors). In the Global Fund's court: Experimentation, evaluation, and the AMFm. *The Lancet* 380(9858). http://www. thelancet.com/journals/lancet/article/PIIS0140-6736(12)62123-0/ fulltext?rss=yes. Accessed on January 20, 2021.

[62] Tougher S, Ye Y, Amuasi JH *et al.* 2012. Effect of the Affordable Medicines Facility — malaria (AMFm) on the availability, price, and market share of quality-assured artemisinin-based combination therapies in seven countries: A before-and-after analysis of outlet survey data. *The Lancet*. 380: 1916–1926. In Bump, J., Fan, Lanthorn, H., Yavuz E. In the Global Fund's court: Experimentation, evaluation, and the AMFm. *The Lancet* 380(9858). http://www.thelancet.com/ journals/lancet/article/PIIS0140-6736(12)62123-0/fulltext?rss=yes. Accessed on January 20, 2021.

[63] Macro International Inc. Global Fund five-year evaluation: Study area 3 — the impact of collective efforts on the reduction of the disease burden of AIDS, tuberculosis and malaria. May, 2009. p. ES-38. http://www.theglobalfund.org/en/terg/ evaluations/5year/. Accessed on August 18, 2016.

[64] Parkhurst J, Ghilardi L, Webster J, Snow R, Lynch CA. Competing interests, clashing ideas and institutionalizing influence: Insights into the political economy of malaria control from seven African countries. *Health Policy and Planning*, czaa166, https://doi.org/10.1093/heapol/czaa166. Accessed on January 26, 2021.

[65] Deaton A. 2013. The Great Escape: Health, Wealth, and the Origins of Inequality. Princeton, Princeton University Press. pp. 267–324.

[66] Alcorn T. 2012. What has the US global health initiative achieved? https:// www.thelancet.com/journals/lancet/article/piis0140-6736(12)61697-3/fulltext. Accessed on January 26, 2021.

[67] National Institute for Health and Care Excellence. https://www.nice.org.uk/ Accessed on May 5, 2021.

[68] Jha P, Jamison DT, Watkins DA, Bell J. 2021. A global compact to counter vaccine nationalism. *The Lancet*. https://doi.org/10.1016/S0140-6736(21)01105-3. Accessed on May 18, 2021.

[69] Owings L. Research colonialism still plagues Africa. https://www.scidev.net/ sub-saharan-africa/scidev-net-investigates/research-colonialism-still-plagues-africa/. Accessed on May 4, 2021.

Chapter 5

Capitalism, Mining, and Restorative Justice in Southern Africa

"The past is never dead. It's not even past."

—William Faulkner[a]

"Don't push me 'cause I'm close to the edge
I'm trying not to lose my head"

— Grandmaster Flash and The Furious Five[b]

It is always a pleasure to hear the words: "Welcome to O. R. Tambo, the international airport in Johannesburg." Once past immigration check ("Welcome, my brother!"), and having traveled light with no checked-in luggage, I was soon on the road to Pretoria. The forum on the mining industry and tuberculosis was intense, substantive, and candid. The brilliant and socially conscious Dr. Yogan Pillay, then Deputy Director-General in the Department of Health of South Africa, was there. During a coffee break, Dr. Barry Kistnasamy (Compensation Commissioner) *remarked that had I arrived a day earlier, I would have witnessed power failure in the area. That was because some people had reportedly stolen*

---

[a]Faulkner W. 2011. *Requiem for a Nun*. New York: Vintage Books. First international edition. p. 73.
[b]Grandmaster Flash and The Furious Five. 1982. *The Message*. https://genius.com/Grandmaster-flash-and-the-furious-five-the-message-lyrics. Accessed on July 27, 2021.

127

parts from a transformer down the road. Such acts were euphemistically called "redistribution" of wealth from the affluent to the poor masses. Clearly, in this nation that Archbishop Desmond Tutu inimitably called The Rainbow People of God, the patience of the poor was wearing thin.

Synopsis

The convergence of capitalism, private enterprise, and public policy provides fascinating and vexing lessons for the practice of global health in the Southern Africa region. Much of the contemporary discourse on health systems focuses on its complex adaptive nature[1-4] or on building blocks.[5] But while such thinking is relevant to the "what" and the "how" of health systems, it does not explain in depth the "why" of health systems. Yet, it is in the interest of country policy makers and investors at the country and global levels to understand why any particular system is the way it is. Such understanding, which explains — but neither justifies nor excuses — apparent irrationalities and clear injustices in health systems, is a precondition for effective leadership in seemingly impossible situations.

This chapter examines a regional challenge: addressing the legacy of unfettered capitalism and state-enforced racism in the mining sector of Southern Africa. It then examines the nascent health financing reforms in one country — the Republic of South Africa itself, with emphasis on the complex social and political dynamics of change and a potential for restorative justice after decades of ruthless exploitation.

5.1. The Mining Industry

South Africa became the single biggest producer of gold within two decades of the initial discovery of that precious mineral on the Witwatersrand in 1886.[6] The mineral wealth that financed industrialization in the country came with significant gains for immigrants and migrant workers from Europe, but it had catastrophic consequences for the indigenous populations. That divergence of fortunes was a deliberate combination of unbridled capitalism and racism whose effects are partly laid bare at the convergence of employment patterns, infections, chronic lung disease, and the post-apartheid inheritance. But first, how was the foundation laid?

Wilson[7] noted that mining shaped the political economy of South Africa in ways that entrenched a system of forced and undulating migrant labor. Black men from all over Southern Africa, not only from within South Africa, were recruited to work the gold mines. They lived in single-sex compounds and were sent home at the end of their contracts. The laws prevented the miners from living near the mines and having their families join them.

From 1906 to 1986, employment in gold mines affiliated with the Chamber of Mines increased from 81,000 to 534,000. By 1986, of the black workers in the mines, 60% were from South Africa, 20% from Lesotho, and the remaining were from Mozambique, Botswana, Malawi, and Eswatini.

Wilson also identified three major consequences to this system of migration. One was economic: the workers' home regions became steadily impoverished because the migrants were not investing their meager wages back home. The second was political. Under apartheid, black men belonged as citizens and husbands in their "homelands." Those homelands became poverty-stricken labor reserves. The rural households, being dependent on the white-controlled apartheid economy, could safely be designated as politically independent. The third consequence was social, based on the plausible origin of the violence of post-apartheid South Africa in the race-driven policy that ensured poverty and forced migration.

The mining system had a two-tier health infrastructure for occupational health services within or near the mines. The upper tier was for white elites in the professional and management categories. The lower tier consisted of small clinics for outpatient services for — mainly black — laborers. However, black mine workers mostly shunned these health facilities because they feared that their illnesses would be reported to their employers, with increased risks of losing their jobs. Thus did the two-tiered system entrench the economic and health gaps between whites and blacks. Furthermore, the apartheid system deepened health and socioeconomic disparities in "homelands," the rural areas that were sources of cheap labor, by systematically under-investing in health infrastructure and basic services. Therefore, the miners were doubly disenfranchised: in mining sites where they had only notional access to primary care despite the occupational hazards, and in their "homelands," which lacked quality health services.

The structure and dynamics of the mining industry in Southern Africa had a fourth, and devastating, consequence in extraordinary dimensions of ill-health, disability, premature deaths, and impoverishment of the miners and their families. That was the foundation for the recent and contemporary experience of interactions between mining, health, and subregional migration in Southern Africa, as detailed by Osewe and Kistnasamy.[8] Migrant mine workers in the subregion face a very high risk burden for silicosis, TB, and HIV/AIDS.[9] The mining sector and its associated cross-border movements of mine workers have amplified the twin epidemics of HIV and TB in the Southern Africa region.[10] The 500,000 mine workers employed in 2,000 mines and quarries across South Africa, of whom about 40% are from Eswatini, Lesotho, and Mozambique, have a TB incidence estimated at 2,500–3,000 per 100,000 persons (the highest in the world), compared to 834 per 100,000 persons in the general population.[11] Chang and colleagues,[12] using two models that integrate diverse types of data, estimated that gold mine workers contribute a disproportionately large number of TB infections in South Africa on a per-capita basis. Thus, the at-risk miners and their families run an additional risk of quantitative invisibility amidst the general population (Box 5.1).

Box 5.1. Separate, Thus Equal: Mining, Apartheid, and Disease in Southern Africa

Working environments in the mining sector, characterized by poor ventilation, high levels of silica exposure, overcrowded housing, and lack of access to appropriate health services, have created a breeding ground for communicable diseases and facilitated the spread of tuberculosis, especially among black mineworkers.[10] These circumstances have been compounded by a legacy of racial differentiation in workers' rights and benefits.[13] Compensation for mineworkers with occupational lung disease was first legislated through the Miner's Phthisis Allowance Act of 1911. Subsequent legislation reflected the ongoing racial inequities, including

(Continued)

Box 5.1. (*Continued*)

differences in medical examinations whereby white mineworkers accessed examinations at the Medical Bureau for Occupational Diseases (MBOD) in central Johannesburg or at one of the subbureaus (Welkom and Witbank) located near the gold mines and coal mines, whereas black mineworkers were examined at the Employment Bureau of Africa (TEBA) offices or mines, where many diseases were missed or not routinely reported to the MBOD. There was also a 12:1 gap in the amount of compensation paid white and black mineworkers, and different forms of compensation were paid to mineworkers suffering from occupational disease — that is, pension payments for white claimants versus differentiated lump sum payments for black claimants.[13,14]

Furthermore, a dual and uneven system of occupational compensation evolved in South Africa — one for mineworkers' lung diseases under the Occupational Diseases in Mines and Works Act, 1973, and one for all other injuries and diseases in all occupations under the Compensation for Occupational Injuries and Diseases Act (COIDA), 1993.[15] This complex system, which essentially created differential benefits for the same occupational lung disease such as silicosis, depending on whether it was acquired through mining or industrial work, has resulted in inferior compensation and benefits for mineworkers.[13] Meanwhile, the system remains complex and difficult to navigate for mineworkers, and for many it has been a significant barrier to accessing compensation.[15] As a result of these challenges, many observers argue that the high disease burden produced within the context of South Africa's mining industry has been a preventable and neglected epidemic.[16]

TB rates in the mining sector in Southern Africa are particularly high because of a convergence of occupational, environmental, and lifestyle-related risk factors. These include exposure to silica dust, cramped living conditions, migration and HIV. For 2019, Lesotho and South Africa were among only five countries in the world with estimated TB incidence of more than 500 cases per 100,000.[17]

Source: Adapted from Osewe PL, Kistnasamy B. 2018. Tuberculosis must fall! : A multisector partnership to address tb in Southern Africa's mining sector. International Development in Focus. Washington, DC: World Bank. https://openknowledge.worldbank.org/handle/10986/30395. Accessed on February 4, 2021.

5.2. Tackling a Wicked Problem

Recent large-scale efforts to tackle the complex problem of TB in the mining industry of Southern Africa involve multiple actors across the private and public sectors at the country, subregional, and global levels. Crucially, getting a more robust understanding of the levers of change underpinned the enterprise. The private sector, which had been seen as the problem (a perception that was wholly justified), became a part of the solution. Building a politically viable coalition around knowledge-based solutions was key to results achieved so far.

The Southern Africa TB Knowledge Hub had several initiatives, key among which was the Southern Africa Mining Sector Initiative.[18] It was conceived as an innovation involving the private and public sectors, civil society, research institutes, associations of ex-miners, labor unions, and development partners to mount a joint effort against TB in the mining sector of the Southern Africa region. Government officials came from Departments of Health, Labor, and Mineral Resources across the region. Coordinated by the World Bank, its scope of work covered studies, consultations, and projects to reduce the incidence of TB in the mines and their surrounding communities. It had three key focus areas: provision of support for better analytical underpinnings for implementation of effective TB interventions; harmonization of treatment protocols and funding to address the challenge (including work on the harmonized management of TB in the mining sector);[19] and innovation and collaboration.

The TB in the Mining Sector Initiative started as a 3-year program to control TB in the mining sector in Lesotho, Mozambique, South Africa, and Eswatini. It aimed to initiate harmonization of TB management in the mining sector across the subregion and to provide proof of concept from which new solutions could emerge.

It is hard to overstate the human dimension of this enterprise, which derives from a combined effect of the harmonization framework for TB diagnosis and treatment, geospatial mapping, continuity of TB care across borders, improved management from diagnosis to treatment, expansion of the One Stop Service Center approach in and beyond South Africa (providing holistic occupational health services and linking mine workers to compensation), review of mine health legislation, improved access to services, and, by mid-2016, tracking and tracing an initial set of about 7,300 mineworkers in five countries. There was progress through demand generation and expanded health infrastructure for occupational health screening in Lesotho, Mozambique, and Eswatini. This was an important change from the situation in 2014, when miners and ex-miners in those countries had to travel long distances to South Africa for screening.

Project-level funding for the work initially came from a US$30 million grant by the GFATM to finance the Southern Africa TB in the Mining Sector Initiative (TIMS). Announced in 2016,[20] the TIMS Project would cover 10 countries in the SADC region. In 2016, the World Bank initially provided US$120 million through the regional Southern Africa TB and Health Systems Strengthening Project in four countries in the SADC region: Lesotho, Mozambique, Zambia and Malawi. In 2020, it announced an additional US$56 million to address Southern Africa's complex TB and HIV epidemics and the closely related occupational lung diseases (OLD).[21,22]

Collaboration between the public and private sectors, especially the mining industry, was essential for the successful launch and continued implementation of this program. The mining industry initially was castigated, with justification, as the source of the problem. That blame was combined with perspectives, eloquently and passionately expressed by some, that the industry should be punished for its part in the health conditions of the miners. After lengthy discussions, key participants converged on the approach of combining private and public capacities to solve the problem of ill-health and missed compensation as swiftly and as comprehensively as possible.

Possibly the most significant development was the Government of South Africa's own domestic financing of a compensation fund. Working across the departments of health, labor, and mineral resources, the government of South Africa initiated a US$100-million program to compensate former mineworkers with compensable lung diseases. A project to track, trace, and register former mineworkers followed. By 2018, it had identified about 100,000 former mineworkers who had been flagged on the database as eligible for compensation.[23] That initiative benefited from the Southern Africa TB in the Mining Sector Initiative's generation of detailed information on the demographic characteristics of current and former mine workers, as well as the availability of TB screening and treatment facilities to effectively coordinate and implement the regional TB response. The database mapped locations and names of all villages in Southern Africa, routes used by mine workers and ex-mine workers, and the nearest health facilities. Enabled by geospatial mapping, it was designed to show migration patterns linked to road networks on a common GPS platform.[24]

5.3. Early Gains

In September 2016, a joint learning session that included Godfrey Oliphant (Deputy Minister for Mineral Resources), Barry Kistnasamy, the managers and operators of a one-stop center and a call center (calling, tracking, tracing, and fielding questions from ex-mineworkers), the representative of the industry group (himself a former CEO of a mining company), officials from Tom Tom (the GPS company, in charge of geo-mapping), met with a few of the direct beneficiaries of the compensation exercise. There were widows of deceased ex-miners and a few chronically ill ex-miners who told their own stories. The sessions underscored two lessons. One was about the profound and lasting effects of historical injustices; the socio-economic consequences of the relationship between the mining industry and workers who were treated as expendable were stunning. If anyone needed proof that the mining industry was truly extractive in the most exploitative sense of the word, there was the proof in ailing flesh and blood. The second lesson was about the possibility of change when policy choices and viable coalitions align with the needs of the marginalized. The parties had moved from an adversarial relationship of about 4 years earlier to a mutually beneficial partnership aimed at solving problems, reaching the poor, and stimulating local economies.

5.4. Financing Universal Health Coverage in South Africa

"Tutu decided he would not mince words with Reagan either. "Your president is in the pits as far as blacks are concerned," he told an American journalist. "I found the speech nauseating…. He sits there like the great big white chief of old [who] can tell us black people that we

don't know what is good for us, the white man knows." With the South
African government killing four-year olds, it was nonsense to describe
freedom fighters, who had used peaceful means to oppose racism for fifty
years before taking up arms, as terrorists. Reagan, Thatcher, and Kohl
were saying to blacks that they were dispensable: "I am quite angry.
I think the west, for my part, can go to hell."

—John Allen, on Desmond Tutu[25]

While the previous section was on the subregion of Southern Africa, this section is about the epic policy dynamics of financing UHC in one country, the Republic of South Africa.

When the apartheid era formally ended in 1994, South Africa inherited a health system with two very different realities. One reality, for the affluent, is financed by private health insurance schemes, which serve the (predominantly white) wealthy people. This private health insurance covers about 16% of the population. The public sector serves the other 84% of the population.[26] The realities were separate by design and unequal; private health insurance coverage generally comes with higher quality than is available in the public sector.

How has South Africa sought to finance its quest for universal coverage amidst this toxic inheritance? The Constitution of the Republic of South Africa stipulates the following as part of its Bill of Rights:[27]

"27. Health care, food, water, and social security

1. Everyone has the right to have access to
   a. health care services, including reproductive health care;
   b. sufficient food and water; and
   c. social security, including, if they are unable to support them-
      selves and their dependants, appropriate social assistance.
2. The state must take reasonable legislative and other measures,
within its available resources, to achieve the progressive realisation
of each of these rights.
3. No one may be refused emergency medical treatment."

Furthermore, the National Health Act 61 of 2003[28] intends:

- *"to provide a framework for a structured uniform health system within the Republic, taking into account the obligations imposed by the Constitution and other laws on the national, provincial and local governments with regard to health services; and*
- *to provide for matters connected therewith."*

South Africa's National Health Insurance (NHI)[29] is designed as a single, publicly financed, and publicly administered fund. It is intended to strategically purchase services with a view to ensuring essential care for all South Africans based on their needs and regardless of their socioeconomic status. Implementation of NHI is based on the need to address structural imbalances in the health system and to reduce the burden of disease, with the following design features of intention: (a) Progressive universalism, (b) Mandatory prepayment of health care, (c) Comprehensive Services, (d) Financial risk protection, (e) Single Fund, (f) Strategic purchaser, (g) Single-payer, and (h) Publicly Administered.

In translating constitutional mandate into policy, and in translating policy into practice, the citizenry, policy makers, private sector investors, and service providers face several questions. There are questions about what constitutes "reasonable legislative and other measures within available resources," and the practical meaning of "progressive realization." There are also questions about the practical realities of a "structured uniform health system" under the constitutionally mandated provisions. These questions are considered in two dimensions: the technocratic on the one hand, and the sociopolitical on the other hand.

5.4.1 Technocratic dimension: Financing, incentives, and functions

South Africa compares favorably with other UMICs in terms of its total health spending, both in Purchasing Power Parity (PPP) terms and as a percentage of GDP, as indicated in Table 5.1.[30] However, like any other health system, resources are finite and demand is potentially infinite, leading to vexing questions about rationing, intra-country redistribution of resources and reframing of social narratives, a complexity that is

Table 5.1.   Health Financing in South Africa

Country Group/ Specific Country	Health Spending per Capita, 2016 (US$)	Health Spending per Capita, 2016 ($PPP)	Health Spending per GDP, 2016 (%)	Government Health Spending per Total Health Spending, 2016 (%)	Out of Pocket Spending per Total Health Spending (%)	DAH per Total Health Spending, 2016 (%)
High income	5,252	5,621	10.8	79.6	13.8	0
Upper-middle income	491	1,009	5.0	53.9	53.9	0.2
Lower-middle income	81	274	3.2	32.1	56.1	3.2
Low income	40	125	5.1	26.3	42.4	25.4
Sub-Saharan Africa	80	199	4.1	36.8	31.5	14.0
South Africa	512	1,162	5.6	53.6	7.8	2.3

Source: Adapted from Global Burden of Disease Health Financing Collaborator Network. 2019. Past, present, and future of global health financing: A review of development assistance, government, out-of-pocket, and other private spending on health for 195 countries, 1995–2050. *The Lancet*, 393: 2233–2260. Published Online April 25, 2019. https://www.thelancet.com/journals/lancet/article/PIIS0140-6736(19)30841-4/fulltext.

sometimes missed by observers who engage in simplistic cheerleading about how easily South Africa could afford NHI.[31] Every health system rations care; the question is whether the rationing is explicit or implicit, and which trade-offs the society is willing and able to live with. Those trade-offs are affected by the structures and instruments of the health finance system. In what might be called the current transition from the inherited system to the desired system, South African health services are financed through general tax revenue, direct OOP, and contributions to private medical insurance. Ataguba and McIntyre,[32] applying standard and innovative methodologies for assessing progressivity, found that general taxes and medical scheme contributions remained progressive, while direct OOP and indirect taxes were regressive. However, private health insurance contributions, across only the insured, were regressive.

Table 5.2.   Intentions and Derailers in South Africa's NHI Reforms

NHI Reform Pillars	Potential Stumbling Blocks
Move beyond the inheritance of fragmented public and private health financing systems	• Private medical schemes as a key stakeholder • People as taxpayers and consumers of health services
Move from voluntary to mandatory prepayment system	• High unemployment
Raise additional revenue for health care	• Lack of trust in public institutions and regressive aspects of VAT • Budgets • Political will is fickle
Improve pooling arrangements so as to better spread risk and improve cross-subsidization	• Independence of medical schemes
Purchase from a mix of public and private providers	• Alleged corruption in the system
Use economies of scale and purchasing methods to achieve cost-efficiency	• Drivers of private health costs
Deliver quality services and continual improvements in health outcomes	• Provincialization instead of district health authorities • Incompetence and failure of leadership and governance at all levels of the health system • High HIV burden and a cocktail of epidemics

Source: Adapted from Michel J, Tediosi F, Egger M, *et al.* 2020. Universal health coverage financing in South Africa: wishes vs. reality. *Journal of Global Health Reports*. 4: e2020061. doi:10.29392/001c.13509. Accessed on February 11, 2021.

The biggest challenges lie in moving from political declaration and legislation to implementation in a situation with a difficult inheritance, and with potential winners and losers all too aware of the stakes. Michel and colleagues[33] provide a very helpful examination of the potential stumbling blocks in the path of NHI reforms. Among the stumbling blocks they identified were those in Table 5.2.

5.4.2 Political dimension: Restorative justice and social engineering

At first glance, the major sociopolitical tension is illustrated by the gaps between intention and execution. South Africa has a clear process for budget formulation from national to provincial governments. But this transparency does not fully apply to decisions on fund allocation from provincial treasuries to health. There are wide interprovince variations in the mechanisms of budget execution. Furthermore, the link between budget process and performance indicators needs strengthening.[34] A closer look reveals that fundamental to South Africa's modest progress toward UHC is a more complex version of what Ichoku and colleagues posit about sub-Saharan Africa: an elitist post-colonial political economy that dominates the social organization in the subregion.[35] Given the inheritance of a dual health infrastructure in which geographic areas with a majority of the country's population are served by relatively mediocre and understaffed health facilities, a key sociopolitical challenge is how to expand quality services to the population. That comes amidst the realities of entrenched resistance from a well-served segment of the population that sees such expansion as a threat to its own legacy of privilege.

The inherited consequences of extractive capitalism and the unbridled racism of apartheid are driving the turmoil in South Africa's quest for UHC. The sweeping reforms envisaged in the NHI require explicit and implicit redistribution of state-conferred legitimacy from a small but wealthy minority to a large and previously subjugated majority. To those who constructed and benefited from the prior situation, that change is a quasi-existential threat.

On the brighter side, the quest for restorative justice is also a beacon of hope. South Africa laid the foundation for a better future via its Truth and Reconciliation Commission.[36] Restorative justice in this context, which has a positive aim that disproportionately favors the previously dispossessed, is not the same as punitive justice, which would aim to serve retribution to the inflictors of pain. It is akin to the practical consequences of Brown versus Board of Education in the United States, which resulted in school desegregation despite organized and often vehement resistance in many places.

5.5. Conclusion

Post-apartheid South Africa could not possibly maintain its inherently unjust legacy of separate and unequal health systems. It cannot afford to create a parallel system for the majority black population that is of the same quality as what the minority affluent white population had under the private health schemes. This point is crucial; in the United States, the underpinning of the strategy that led to the Brown versus Board of Education victory was that the states could not afford to set up a parallel system of equal quality to those previously reserved for whites only. Charles Houston, who taught and guided Thurgood Marshall in that epic legal struggle, approached the challenge as a matter of social engineering.[37] The NHI and its associated reforms in South Africa constitute the foundation for medium- to long-term social engineering. Warts and all, perhaps the only politically viable scenario is a unified system in which the public sector and the private sector play complementary roles to achieve public policy goals. The reforms could eventually achieve substantial success, albeit with imperfections.

References

[1] Lipsitz L. 2012. Understanding health care as a complex system: The foundation for unintended consequences. *JAMA*, 308(3): 243–244. https://www.ncbi.nlm.nih.gov/pmc/articles/PMC3511782/. Accessed on February 13, 2021.

[2] Plsek P. 2001. Redesigning health care with insights from the science of complex adaptive systems. In *Crossing the Quality Chasm: A New Health System for the 21st Century*. Washington DC: The National Academies Press. p. 13.

[3] Martínez-García M, Hernández-Lemus M. 2013. Health systems as complex systems. *American Journal of Operations Research*, 3 (1A): Article ID:27538, 14 pages. https://www.scirp.org/html/5-1040216_27538.htm?pagespeed=noscript. Accessed on February 13, 2021.

[4] Paina L, Peters DH. 2012. Understanding pathways for scaling up health services through the lens of complex adaptive systems. *Health Policy and Planning*, 27(5): 365–373. https://academic.oup.com/heapol/article/27/5/365/751682. Accessed on February 13, 2021.

[5] World Health Organization. 2007. Everybody's business: strengthening health systems to improve health outcomes. WHO's Framework for Action. Geneva:

World Health Organization. https://www.who.int/healthsystems/strategy/en/. Accessed on February 13, 2021.

[6] Richardson P, van Helten J. 1984. The Development of the South African Gold-Mining Industry, 1895–1918. *The Economic History Review*, 37(3): 319–340. https://doi.org/10.2307/2597284. https://www.jstor.org/stable/2597284.

[7] Wilson F. 2001. Minerals and migrants: how the mining industry has shaped South Africa. *Daedalus,* 130(1), Why South Africa matters, Winter, 99–121. https://www.jstor.org/stable/20027681?read-now=1&seq=10#page_scan_tab_contents Accessed on February 1, 2021.

[8] Osewe, Patrick L, Kistnasamy, Barry. 2018. *Tuberculosis Must Fall!: A Multisector Partnership to Address TB in Southern Africa's Mining Sector. International Development in Focus.* Washington, DC: World Bank. https://open-knowledge.worldbank.org/handle/10986/30395. Accessed on February 4, 2021.

[9] Rosenstock L, Cullen M, Fingerhut M. 2006. Occupational health. In *Disease Control Priorities in Developing Countries*, 2d ed., edited by D. T. Jamison *et al.* Washington, DC: World Bank; New York: Oxford University Press.

[10] Stuckler D, Basu S, McKee M. 2010. Governance of mining, HIV, and tuberculosis in Southern Africa. *Global Health Governance*, 4(1). http://www.ghgj.org/Stuckler_final.pdf. Accessed on February 12, 2021.

[11] Lebina L, Martinson N, Milovanovic M, A. Kinghorn A. 2013. TB, HIV and silicosis in miners: epidemiological data on tuberculosis, multi-drug resistant TB, silicosis and HIV among miners and ex-miners in Southern Africa. In Osewe, Patrick L; Kistnasamy, Barry. 2018. *Tuberculosis Must Fall!: A Multisector Partnership to Address TB in Southern Africa's Mining Sector.* International Development in Focus. Washington, DC: World Bank. https://openknowledge. worldbank.org/handle/10986/30395. p. 14. Accessed on February 12, 2021.

[12] Chang ST, Chihota VN, Fielding KL, Grant AD, Houben RM, White RG, Churchyard GJ, Eckhoff PA, Wagner BG. 2018. Small contribution of gold mines to the ongoing tuberculosis epidemic in South Africa: a modeling-based study. *BMC Medicine*, 16(52). https://bmcmedicine.biomedcentral.com/articles/10.1186/s12916-018-1037-3.

[13] Ehrlich, R. 2012. A century of miners' compensation in South Africa. *American Journal of Industrial Medicine*, 55: 560–569.

[14] Nelson, G. 2013. Occupational respiratory diseases in the South African mining industry. *Global Health Action*, 6. http://doi.org/10.3402/gha.v6i0.19520.

[15] Naidoo RN. 2013. Mining: South Africa's legacy and burden in the context of occupational respiratory diseases. *Global Health Action*, 6: 20512. http://dx.doi.org/10.3402/gha.v6i0.20512.

[16] Roberts J. 2009. The *Hidden Epidemic Amongst Former Miners: Silicosis, Tuberculosis and the Occupational Diseases in Mines and Works Act in the Eastern Cape, South Africa*. Durban: Health Systems Trust.

[17] World Health Organization. 2020. *Global Tuberculosis Report 2020*. p. 33. https://www.who.int/teams/global-tuberculosis-programme/data. Accessed on February 12, 2021.

[18] World Bank. The Southern Africa TB in the mining sector initiative. https://www.worldbank.org/en/programs/the-southern-africa-tb-in-the-mining-sector-initiative#1. Accessed on February 7, 2021.

[19] Framework for the harmonized management of tuberculosis in the mining sector. http://pubdocs.worldbank.org/en/815231483123459059/Framework-for-the-Harmonized-Management-of-Tuberculosis-in-the-Mining-Sector. Accessed on March 12, 2021.

[20] GFATM. 2016. Grant to fight TB in Southern Africa's mining sector. https://www.theglobalfund.org/en/news/2016-02-05-grant-to-fight-tb-in-southern-africa-s-mining-sector/. Accessed on February 7, 2021.

[21] World Bank. 2020. Scaling up support to help combat tuberculosis and occupational lung diseases in Southern Africa. https://www.worldbank.org/en/news/press-release/2020/06/19/scaling-up-support-to-help-combat-tuberculosis-and-occupational-lung-diseases-in-southern-africa. Accessed February 8, 2021.

[22] World Bank. 2020. Lesotho, Malawi, Eastern, Central and Southern Africa Health Community, and Africa Union Development Agency — New partnership for Africa development — Southern Africa Tuberculosis and Health Systems Support Project: Additional financing (English). https://projects.worldbank.org/en/projects-operations/document-detail/P173228. Accessed on February 8, 2021.

[23] Osewe PL, Kistnasamy B. 2018. *Tuberculosis Must Fall!: A Multisector Partnership to Address TB in Southern Africa's Mining Sector*. International Development in Focus. Washington, DC: World Bank. https://openknowledge.worldbank.org/handle/10986/30395. Accessed on February 4, 2021.

[24] World Bank. 2017. The Southern Africa TB in the mining sector initiative. https://www.worldbank.org/en/programs/the-southern-africa-tb-in-the-mining-sector-initiative#4. Accessed on February 10, 2021.

[25] Desmond Tutu AJ. 2006. *Rabble Rouser for Peace*. Chicago, IL: Lawrence Hill Books. pp. 260–261.

[26] Health Policy Project. Health Financing Profile. South Africa. 2016. https://www.healthpolicyproject.com/pubs/7887/SouthAfrica_HFP.pdf. Accessed on June 8, 2021.

[27] Constitution of the Republic of South Africa, 1996 — Chapter 2: bill of rights. https://www.gov.za/documents/constitution/chapter-2-bill-rights#27. Accessed on February 10, 2021.

[28] Government of South Africa. National Health Act 61 of 2003. https://www.gov.za/documents/national-health-act. Accessed on February 11, 2021.

[29] Government of South Africa. Department of Health. National Health Act, 2003. National health insurance coverage. Towards universal health coverage. Number 627. Government Gazette, June 30, 2017. https://www.gov.za/documents/national-health-act-national-health-insurance-policy-towards-universal-health-coverage-30. Accessed on February 10, 2021.

[30] Global Burden of Disease Health Financing Collaborator Network. 2019. Past, present, and future of global health financing: a review of development assistance, government, out-of-pocket, and other private spending on health for 195 countries, 1995–2050. *The Lancet*, 393: 2233–2260. Published Online April 25, 2019. https://www.thelancet.com/journals/lancet/article/PIIS0140-6736(19)30841-4/fulltext. Accessed on February 12, 2021.

[31] Yates R. South Africa can easily afford national health insurance. https://www.chathamhouse.org/2019/12/south-africa-can-easily-afford-national-health-insurance. Accessed on February 11, 2021.

[32] Ataguba JE, McIntyre D. 2018. The incidence of health financing in South Africa: findings from a recent data set. *Health Economics, Policy and Law*, 13(1): 68–91. https://doi.org/10.1017/S1744133117000196. Accessed on February 11, 2021.

[33] Michel J, Tediosi F, Egger M, *et al.* 2020. Universal health coverage financing in South Africa: Wishes vs reality. *Journal of Global Health Reports*, 4: e2020061. doi:10.29392/001c.13509. Accessed on February 11, 2021.

[34] James C, Gemeinder M, Rivadeneira A, Vammalle C. 2018. Health financing and budgeting practices for health in South Africa. *OECD Journal on Budgeting*, 95–126. https://doi.org/10.1787/budget-17-5j8sd88t3sr3. Accessed on February 11, 2021

[35] Ichoku HE, Fonta WM, Ataguba JE. 2012. Political Economy and History: Making Sense of health financing in Sub-Saharan Africa. *Journal of International Development*. https://doi.org/10.1002/jid.2842. Accessed on February 11, 2021.

[36] Truth and Reconciliation Commission. 1998. The report of the Truth and Reconciliation Commission. https://www.justice.gov.za/trc/report/index.htm. Accessed on February 12, 2021.

[37] James R. 2010. *Root and Branch: Charles Hamilton Houston, Thurgood Marshall, and the Struggle to End Segregation*. Bloomsbury Press, 1st edition.

Chapter 6

Investing, Transitions, and Disease Control in Russia

"Russia is not a country that can be kept waiting in the ante-room."

"Amerìkānskī! Angliyskiy! Come with me! I know Hollywood!" The banging on the door was loud and insistent. I woke up, startled, and wondered what was happening. Bang! Bang! "Amerìkānskī! Angliyskiy! Come with me! I know Hollywood!" It was the middle of a very cold winter night, on a 13-hour train journey from Moscow to Cheboksary, the capital of Chuvashia, a federal subject of Russia. The train had left Moscow right on schedule. We had stopped around midnight at a small town where middle-aged women held ornate chandeliers up to our windows, seeking to sell them at seemingly give-away prices. Those beautiful chandeliers were tempting, but carrying them back to Washington DC would be clumsy. I passed. But why were they selling chandeliers around midnight, in the middle of nowhere? Someone speculated that they were factory workers who had been paid in kind in a demonetized local economy; the chandeliers were their salaries.

---

[a]Llyod J. 1998. *Rebirth of a Nation: An Anatomy of Russia*. London: Michael Joseph. p. 356.

My colleague, with whom I shared a cubicle with a double bunk bed in the train, also woke up because of the loud noise. He was puzzled. After a quick huddle, we concluded that the man at the door, perhaps under the influence of too much vodka,[1] had assumed that foreigners in these parts must be thrill-seeking American and English tourists and was just rambling about Hollywood because he had seen too many American movies of the tacky variety. Any aspirations we had for acting careers in Hollywood would have to wait for real talent scouts, as would any restroom break in the hours that remained on the journey. The would-be Hollywood agent soon went away and the rest of the journey was uneventful.

Synopsis

This chapter unpacks the dynamics of science, politics, and controversies around investing in tuberculosis (TB) and HIV/AIDS control in the Russian Federation, following its emergence from the Soviet era. The challenge was to successfully negotiate with Russia an agreement to combine technical guidelines from the World Health Organization (WHO) with financing from an external multilateral development financier — the World Bank — for a large program to curb the dual epidemics of TB and HIV/AIDS. The chapter begins with an overview of the context of political and economic transition from the Soviet Union to the Russian Federation and an overview of TB and HIV/AIDS in Russia. This is followed by deeper dives into the logic of development assistance for the health sector — and specifically for disease control — in Russia and a closer examination of the HIV/AIDS problem. Attention then turns to the challenges of learning, adapting, and scaling. This is followed by an exploration of how the impasse around foreign investment in the program was resolved through complex transactions and bargaining that informed the agreement between Russia and international institutions.

6.1. The Political and Economic Transitions

Starting in the early 1990s, multiple upheavals nudged Russia to rethink its long-established health system, including the compact between the

State and its citizens, financing, service delivery, public health, disease control, learning, and relationships with other countries and non-Russian institutions. The decisions driving those changes in the health system are arguably best understood within the broader historic and socio-political narrative of the country at that time.

The Soviet Union was officially dissolved in December 1991 and Mikhail Gorbachev resigned the presidency that same month.[2] Those events created a major convergence of tensions that led to changes in the health system. The formerly socialist countries of Central and Eastern Europe that sought accession to the EU hoped to achieve higher living standards and more individual freedom.[3] By contrast, while Russia sought a political break from its Soviet past, higher living standards, and greater individual freedom, there was neither Russian interest in nor an obvious pathway to EU accession. Its socio-political transition was a cataclysmic exercise in muddling through.

The epic tensions of the transition impacted the health system. Although the USSR *de jure* guaranteed health services for everyone, the reality was different. In post-Soviet Russia, the gap between declarations of abundance and reality of shortages became a chasm in the early years of the Federation, compounded by inflation and continuing economic decline. Measures of health service infrastructure, such as hospital beds per capita, became markers of a bloated system when compared to the OECD countries. The fragmentation of a previously centralized command-and-control system degraded the public health surveillance and disease control system. Having lost the halo of its superpower status, Russia found itself in an unfamiliar situation of having to reckon with the perspectives and preferences of external technical advisors and financiers.

6.2. Tuberculosis and HIV/AIDS in Immediate Post-Soviet Russia

Russia's response to its syndemic of TB and HIV/AIDS illustrates how the country and external actors navigated the challenge of health system reform during the transition from socialism to a semblance of a market economy.

Before the break-up of the USSR, the prevention and treatment of TB were under strict federal control. That command was weakened following the collapse of the USSR, causing the degradation of TB control in Russia.[4] Domestic financing of TB control declined. Workers were demoralized. Drug-resistant strains of *Mycobacterium tuberculosis,* a bacterium that causes TB, emerged. Cases and deaths from TB increased. It was especially bad in the prison system, where the registration rate among prisoners was 4,347 per 100,000 in 1999, and made up 25% of all new TB cases in the country.[5] Of the 300,000 people released from the prisons during that period, 30,000 were estimated to have had active TB, and at least 10,000 of those 30,000 probably had multidrug-resistant TB. Therefore, the prisons were regarded as an epidemiological pump that drove increased TB incidence and prevalence in the general population.[6] There is a Yoruba proverb that translates as "there is dignity in togetherness, as long as we are not in prison." Having visited a Russian prison in the privileged position of a World Bank staff working on health, I can attest to the wisdom of that proverb.

Box 6.1 provides a summary of TB control amidst the transition in Russia, where the concurrent problem of HIV, the virus that causes AIDS, added to the TB challenge. In 1986, the year before the first official case of HIV was formally registered in Russia, a Soviet health official named Vladimir Trofimov portrayed the new disease as a Western problem. There was no home for it in Russia he reportedly said, "since in Russia there is no drug addiction and no prostitution."[9] Such denial did not prepare Russia to effectively confront what was unfolding.

WHO and UNAIDS reported that Eastern Europe and Central Asia had the world's fastest-growing HIV/AIDS epidemic in 2002 (Figure 6.1), with an estimated 250,000 new infections and 1.2 million people living with HIV/AIDS.[10] It was a fast-growing problem in Russia and most of the infections initially were among injecting drug users (IDUs). But it would not remain confined to that especially high-risk group. The risk was high of HIV transmission from IDUs to their sex partners, some of whom were also Commercial Sex Workers. Those would serve as a bridge for HIV to spread into the general population. A study in Togliatti City was especially insightful.[11]

Box 6.1. Transition and the TB Control System in Russia

While Russia embarked on a transition from the centrally planned Soviet economy to a more open society and a rather poorly regulated market economy, its TB control system remained the same, with institutional reluctance to change. Information on TB prevalence and treatment impact was classified information during Soviet times. The approach to TB control was costly because it was overly reliant on mass screenings, often along professional groups by X-rays for diagnosis (the so-called fluoroscopy), lengthy hospitalizations for treatment, and frequent use of surgery. The power of the Federal Government to enforce compliance with these screening programs that target non-symptomatic population groups had diminished, rendering these expensive programs largely ineffective.

Nonetheless, the Soviet approach to TB control was held in high esteem by the Russian health establishment, partly because the TB burden in the late Soviet era was not the big problem that it became in the 1990s, according to the official data. An exception was the Ministry of Justice, which had expressed its willingness to use internationally recognized guidelines to manage the huge TB problem among prisoners. This willingness became possible after the prison health service was transferred from the Ministry of Interior to the Ministry of Justice as part of overall judicial reform in Russia. However, while the Ministry of Justice ran a parallel system of TB control services, its desire for change was contingent upon endorsement by the Ministry of Health. In addition, the incentives for financing the TB services favored the maintenance of large TB hospitals and sanatoria because they were based on the number of beds. Such an input-driven system does not help to improve performance based on outcomes. Furthermore, a generation of practitioners, distinguished in the Soviet era, resisted rapid change from the familiar system to the new one. As a result, promising approaches remained in the pilot phase, on a scale at which they could not be perceived to threaten the established order.

Russia also had an epidemic of multidrug-resistant TB (MDR-TB) that was caused by strains of the TB bacteria that were resistant to at least isoniazid and rifampicin, the two principal first-line drugs used in combination chemotherapy. MDR-TB results from poor management of drug-sensitive TB; it was a big problem caused by a failure to manage a

(Continued)

Box 6.1. (*Continued*)

smaller problem effectively. It was the result of one or more of the multiple
failures in the disease control or the broader health care system.

In cross-country comparisons, the MDR rate among previously
untreated cases was inversely correlated with treatment success under short-
course chemotherapy (SCC).[7] The straightforward conclusion was that
high cure rates had prevented the emergence of resistance in countries that
made effective use of SCC. If few patients failed treatment, fewer still could
develop resistance. High rates of resistance tended to be associated with low
treatment success. In Ivanovo Oblast, Russia, the reported treatment success for patients carrying fully sensitive strains was 63%; with a cure rate
this low, it was not surprising that 9% of new TB cases are MDR.[8] MDR-TB
was perceived as a growing hazard to human health worldwide.[6]

Source: Adeyi O, Fidler A, Gracheva M, Loginova T. 2003/2004.
Tuberculosis and AIDS control in Russia: Closing the knowing-doing gap.
Eurohealth, 9(4) Winter. https://www.lse.ac.uk/lse-health/assets/documents/
eurohealth/issues/eurohealth-v9n4.pdf. Accessed on June 18, 2021.

There were growing concerns that official data seriously underesti-
mated the scale and speed of the HIV/AIDS problem in Russia. Yet,
instead of mobilizing a strong and robust response to HIV/AIDS, the
Russian health establishment was mired in a mixture of officious denial
and lethargy. This inaction, which at first glance was baffling to outsiders,
derived from a combination of several factors. The epidemic at that time
was being driven by the spread of HIV among IDUs in the prison system.
IDUs thus constituted a group of high-risk core transmitters; curbing the
spread of HIV required interruption of transmission among IDUs and
from IDUs via *bridge groups* (the sexual partners of IDUs) to the general
population. However, the *sotto voce* Russian position was that since the
use (including intravenously) of narcotic drugs was illegal in Russia, there
was no such drug use in the prisons, and hence there was no need for
interventions to prevent HIV spread among IDUs. While this circular

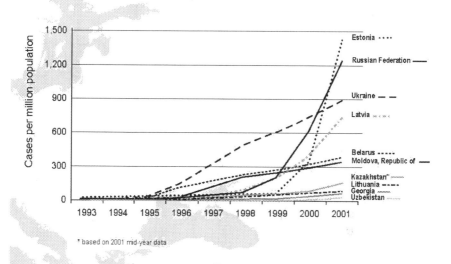

Figure 6.1. Cumulative Reported HIV Infections per Million Population, Eastern European Countries: 1993–2001

Source: European Center for the Epidemiological Monitoring of AIDS. HIV/AIDS surveillance in Europe. End-year report 2001. Saint-Maurice. Institut de Veille Sanitaire, 2001. No. 66.

reasoning initially baffled external technical experts, including those from WHO, UNAIDS, and the World Bank, it was truly infuriating for the marginalized Russian NGOs who knew how much damage such institutionalized denial could cause. Anya Sarang, the forthright leader of the Russian Harm Reduction Network at the time, found the official inaction especially frustrating.

6.3. Multidimensional Challenges of Development Assistance for TB and HIV/AIDS Control in Russia

External technical and financing agencies operated on an implicit assumption that curbing TB and HIV/AIDS in Russia would, in principle, be no more difficult than in other countries with extensive disease control infrastructure, track records of infectious disease control, and strengths in the basic sciences. Therefore, the external expectations could be described in three interrelated pathways to solve the technical problem, as described in Box 6.1. Efforts would need to be focused on ensuring the following:

- technical consistency with the state of the art in global approaches to TB and HIV/AIDS control;
- resource optimization to ensure that Russia got the best value for its own domestic budget;
- learning, adaptation, and scaling.

6.3.1 Convergence with global approaches

Professor Lee Reichman gave a vivid account of the TB control dynamics in Russia during the 1990s in *Timebomb: The Global Epidemic of Multi-Drug-Resistant Tuberculosis*.[6] The book concluded with Russia's rejection of a World Bank loan to fund a large program of TB control and cited a *Financial Times* story by Andrew Jack, dated June 8, 2001:

> *"The Russian government has blocked a $150 million World Bank loan for the treatment of tuberculosis and AIDS, triggering fears of a collapse in health funding within the country at a time of growing concern over a TB epidemic and in increase in HIV infection. The loan, which was requested by the Russian government, has been unexpectedly stalled by the Ministry of Health in a clash over treatment methods and World Bank demands for competitive tender for TB drugs."*

Why did Russia turn down the loan in mid-2001? Reichman noted three contributory factors. First, Russian TB experts did not want to change from their Soviet-era approaches to the WHO-led international standards for treating TB. Second, there was an element of official denial of the scale of the problem. Not only was the prevalence of TB either unknown or deliberately underreported during the Soviet era, but the Russian TB leadership claimed that the scale of the problem was overstated and the country could deal with it on its own; ergo, why borrow money for a small problem? Finally, Russian pride was at stake; their calculus was that preserving Russian *pride* was worth forgoing the financing and technical assistance needed to fix their disastrous TB problem, which was already spreading to the West.

Reichman's observations were correct but incomplete. They did not include some of the nuance and realpolitik that explained Russia's *seemingly* irrational obstinacy.

There was a gap between the Russian narrative and external expectations of immediate gratification in arriving at *technical convergence with the state of the art in global approaches to TB and HIV/AIDS control.* Little in the traditional DAH approaches to technical assistance, program preparation, and multi-agency financing coalitions prepared external institutions to successfully manage their engagement with Russia.

Many external parties came into Russia with a faulty logic, the lessons of which were deep and painful. The expectations of external agencies centered around the demonstrated effectiveness of Directly Observed Therapy-Short Course (DOTS) for treating TB, and of the DOTS-Plus regimen for treating MDR-TB in Tomsk, Siberia. Although the Tomsk Project complied with the standard evidence-based regimen used in industrialized countries and in many developing countries, it was very different from the treatment approved by the Russian Ministry of Health.

The Ministry of Finance had the final say in matters of external financing. But it would not approve a loan for the health sector unless the relevant line ministries sought its approval. The Deputy Head of the MOF's International Cooperation and External Debt Management, Alexander Pavlov, was implacably opposed to the potential World Bank loan. Nothing moved past his desk and no reason was given for seemingly interminable delays in making apparently simple decisions by his office.

While the Ministry of Justice, charged with healthcare provision in the prison system, expressed interest in a large program to curb the TB and HIV/AIDS epidemics in prisons, this was not the case with the Ministry of Health, which exercised overall leadership of the health sector. Indeed, in mid-2001, the Ministry of Health was feeling disrespected by non-Russian institutions on three fronts: NGOs working in Tomsk Region, the WHO, and the World Bank. At first glance, WHO was simply doing its job as the global guardian of standards in public health in treating drug-sensitive TB. However, as detailed by Lee Reichman, WHO fell very short in its initial approaches to MDR-TB, since it quietly took a position that amounted to giving up on those with MDR-TB.[6] The World Bank was interested in supporting large-scale reform of Russia's antiquated TB control system. In an important signal, contrary to standard practice elsewhere, the leader of the WHO mission to Russia was not called a WHO Representative (WR) but was designated as The Special Envoy of the WHO Director-General to the Russian Federation. The *cognoscenti* knew the reason: if there was no WR in the United States, why should Russia, which saw itself as a power equal to the United States, have a WR? In the autumn of 2001, posters on the corridor leading to the ministerial conference room of the MOH castigated unspecified external agencies that neither understood nor respected Russia.

Worse still, the most prominent Russian TB experts felt insulted and humiliated by the perceived arrogance and swashbuckling approach of Westerners in the pilot project in Tomsk. In September 2001, Academician Professor Mikhail Perelman, Director of the Research Institute for Phthisiopulmonology and Chief Phthisiologist of the Russian Ministry of Health, met with Julian Schweitzer (then World Bank Country Director for Russia) and me. I had just taken on responsibility as the World Bank's Team Leader for the controversial and moribund TB and AIDS Program. My responsibilities were to avert a disaster, build trust with a vexed superpower, and save the program — no pressure!

Perelman, simultaneously soft spoken and acerbic, maintained that surgery was the proper method for treating TB. This was contrary to WHO's DOTS regimen. Perelman was a Soviet-era pioneer of cardiac and thoracic surgery. He asserted that Russian TB treatment regimens were superior to those being proposed by WHO, upon which the World Bank would finance the TB component of the potential project that had been rejected. Besides, he claimed, the Western experts working on MDR-TB in Tomsk were triumphalist and arrogant. Therefore, Perelman declared, the World Bank should forget about any TB project that would expand the pilot project from Tomsk to all of Russia; it would never happen. Perelman's approach was reminiscent of Andrei Gromyko, the former Soviet Foreign Minister and later President, of whom the *Los Angeles Times* wrote: "With his remarkable memory and mastery of the historical record, he often tried to wear down the other side and win concessions by sheer persistence."[12]

Perelman's approach reflected the *wounded pride* of the Russian TB Establishment. Despite technically rational expectations that the Russians would switch to DOTS and DOTS-Plus on the inherent merit of their clinical effectiveness, well-intentioned Europeans and North Americans misread the social narrative upon which Russia would make its decision. This was a country that prided itself on being the entity that broke the Nazi Third Reich and won the Second World War, which the Russians call the Great Patriotic War. To Russians, Western celebrations of Victory Day in Europe appeared as revisionist hype designed to take credit for a victory which, in their view, was clearly and solely won by the Soviet Union. It was hard for the intellectual elite of Russia to reconcile the status of their country as a great military and cosmonautic power with its reality of ineffectiveness in controlling the growing epidemics of TB and HIV/AIDS.

I had seen similar dynamics play out between western purveyors of development assistance and government officials in other countries. It was especially striking during the war in Ethiopia, which ended in 1991. I had worked for the WHO in Ethiopia. The median technical expert from the Global North looked at Ethiopian officials and saw needy citizens of a poor country. The median Ethiopian looked in the mirror and saw a descendant of those who won the Battle of Adwa — on top of the historical glow of association with the Queen of Sheba and King Solomon. When discussions did not go well, and host country officials felt imposed upon, the median Ethiopian would calmly and confidently tell the *farangi*[b] to go to hell. On my very first day in Ankara, a senior official in the Turkish health sector had pulled me aside after a group dinner during which I had said little other than greetings. He proceeded to share some nuggets. I recall his exact words in that first meeting: "I am happy to meet you. Let me give you some advice. We are the descendants of the Ottoman Empire and we will never do anything that we don't really want to do." He was sharing the mother lode of successful client engagement in DAH: know and understand the narrative of your client, even — or especially — when you differ with them on the basis of strategic logic and technical information. Those experiences in Ethiopia, Turkey, and elsewhere came in useful in Russia; it was essential to combine strategic

---

[b] Foreigner in Amharic.

purpose and technical rigor with attention to the socio-political narrative of the host country as understood by the nationals.

By the summer of 2001, there was practically no working relationship at the policy level between the Russian Ministry of Health and the World Bank. The Russian MOH had expelled from a meeting a highly conscientious and diligent World Bank staff who was based in the Moscow office of the World Bank. Frustrated by Russian foot-dragging, World Bank President Jim Wolfensohn told an interviewer: "I don't much care whether they take our money or somebody else's. My only concern is that action is taken, and I will make a nuisance of myself until that happens."[13]

6.3.2 Value for money

During the earlier iteration of project preparation, the World Bank's team had sought options for international competitive bidding that would enable Russia to access quality-assured TB drugs based on criteria set by WHO and the Green Light Committee of the Stop TB Partnership. This was objectively in Russia's best technical and financial interests: quality, value for money, and transparency. However, Russian manufacturers of pharmaceuticals perceived an existential threat to their commercial viability because those requirements for quality-assured medicines would bring competitors to their domestic market. They mounted a political assault on the project via both the MOH and the Russian Duma (parliament). *The Washington Post* reported this aspect of Russian lobbying on May 8, 2001:[14]

> *"Russia has thrown up unexpected objections to a new $150 million World Bank loan that would be the bank's most ambitious effort yet to combat a rise of epidemic proportions in tuberculosis cases here.*
>
> *In an apparent reversal that one Western critic called 'medical jingoism,' the Health Ministry withdrew its backing for the loan last month. Echoing the arguments of lobbyists for Russia's pharmaceutical industry, the ministry argued that the loan would mainly constitute a boon for Western drugmakers at the expense of local manufacturers.*
>
> *The proposed loan would add significant resources to the Russian government's current $600 million, five-year war on tuberculosis, a*

problem that has grown dramatically in the decade since the Soviet Union's collapse and is now being exacerbated by an accelerating AIDS epidemic that leaves immune-deficient patients more vulnerable to TB."

One concept that did not initially gain traction with the Russian health leadership was cost-effectiveness. This extended beyond the TB and AIDS sphere to the broader systemic consultations on health financing, service delivery, and public health. The primary reason was not a lack of technical understanding. For example, during one especially insightful discussion about allocative efficiency, technical efficiency, and cost-effectiveness, the otherwise well-informed Russian counterparts declared that their priority was to acquire top-line diagnostic and therapeutic equipment so that they would establish parity with the United States, after which they would be ready to talk about reforming their health system and service delivery based on cost-effectiveness. *How would you feel if Russia had won the cold war and Russians were now visiting Chicago to tell Americans what to do?* In matters of health systems in Russia, value, like beauty, lay in the eyes of the beholder.

6.3.3 Learning, adapting, and scaling

Russian leadership thrived on certainty: parameters were fixed and edicts came via the seemingly immutable *Prikaz(es)* orders. Learning and adaptation implicitly conveyed weakness. The "assistance" in Technical Assistance was an insult. This tied the hands of the relatively curious and more open-minded technocrats who were not opposed to forming viable coalitions with external counterparts from bilateral agencies (e.g., CIDA, DFID, USAID) and multilateral agencies (e.g., UNAIDS, WHO, and the World Bank). One such technocrat was Vadim Pokrovsky, the head of the Federal Research Center for AIDS Prevention and Control in Moscow, who was unusually willing to buck the pattern of denial and obfuscation on the growing scourge of HIV/AIDS in Russia. However, the pace of work was plodding and lacked the dynamism needed for building coalitions that would move swiftly and effectively. Outside the government, Anya Sarang, who ably led the Russian Harm Reduction Network, was central to a growing, if officially despised and marginalized, effort to bring harm reduction to the mainstream of HIV/AIDS control in the country. Within Russia, they constituted two nodes of a learning enterprise.

For both diseases — TB and HIV/AIDS, the difficulties that external agencies encountered in securing government consent for small-scale experimentation (as in Tomsk for TB) paled in comparison to the systemic challenge of reaching agreements to invest additional domestic and external resources in large-scale programs. By the end of 2001, DOTS had covered just 12% of the population through about 19 demonstration projects in Russia.[15] The scale was too small and the pace was too slow.

While small-scale efforts in HIV/AIDS prevention and control were intense, they rarely threatened the established order across the 11 time zones of Russia. As such, they could either be humored as the harmless antics of a few amusingly crazy foreigners or snuffed out with little upheaval if the foreign protagonists made too many waves. There was a need for large programs of targeted, non-stigmatizing prevention,[16] combined with serological and behavioral surveillance (the so-called second generation surveillance).[17,18]

With respect to TB, WHO convened a High-Level Working Group (HLWG) that coordinated effort across the pilot projects that were supported by a number of international agencies. The HLWG served as an advisor to update Russia's TB protocols in line with contemporary approaches and WHO guidelines.[19] However, as Reichman noted, even when a new approach to TB control was more effective than an established practice, its countrywide adaptation might be blocked if it did not originate from the "establishment."[6]

In sum, a robust countrywide program on TB and HIV/AIDS threatened the established order; the best way to ensure it never happened was to kill it before it had any chance of being approved by the Russian Federation's government in Moscow. It was a three-dimensional chess game at which the guardians of orthodoxy in TB control and denial of HIV/AIDS in Russia were grandmasters — and they were playing on their home territory. How would the small-scale learning within Russia and external expertise coalesce to enable change on a large scale?

6.4. The Gambit

As we saw, the root cause of the impasse did not lie in technical disagreements about approaches to TB and HIV/AIDS control. It lay in a strategic error. While foreign development and health experts, predominantly from European and North American institutions (including multilateral agencies, bilateral agencies, academia, and NGOs), saw Russians as people who needed to be helped, they failed to engage with the Russians in ways that acknowledged how Russians saw themselves — as citizens of a great power, to be treated with respect, never mind the loss of the cold war.

My colleagues and I understood that Russia had a unique combination of features that complicated decision-making in the health system beyond what was usual elsewhere in the world. It had geopolitical status through its membership of the (now defunct) Group of Eight highly industrialized countries (G8) and its permanent membership of the United Nations Security Council. But it also had high burdens of TB and HIV/AIDS that were more common in LICs and MICs without global clout. Its Soviet legacy did not fit with modern, science-based approaches to infectious disease control. These features severely constrained prospects for large-scale implementation of evidence-based disease control measures.[20]

In hindsight, the risk of the debacle of mid-2001 should have been obvious to technical experts, especially those from Europe and North America, had they internalized the history of empires and the desires of defeated parties to save face. After all, despite no longer having an empire to rule, the British still confer on people honors such as Knight Commander of the British Empire, a practice that is clearly anachronistic and arguably delusional. And despite its futility, the United States repeatedly doubled down on its war in Vietnam, a classic example of the escalation of commitment bias. Similarly, Russia was demonstrating a brew of nostalgia for the glory days of its empire via commitment to inappropriate approaches to TB and HIV/AIDS, the health consequences be damned. It was the Russian version of a *lost cause*, such as the myth that Southern whites of the Confederate States of America clung to in an analgesic effort to rationalize the catastrophic reality of their loss in a campaign into which they had swaggered. James Patterson notes as follows:

> *"In this use, the word 'myth' is not synonymous with 'falsehood' (though it may incorporate many untruths) but rather to be understood in its anthropological meaning as the collective memory of a people about their past, which sustains a belief system that shapes their view of the world in which they live."*[21]

6.4.1 Resolving the impasse

My colleagues and I summarized our first-hand experience in 2003.[20] This section provides more detailed insight.[c] After the debacle of mid-2001, complex, low-decibel consultations resumed in September 2001 across multiple aspects of the health system in Russia, including but not limited to TB and HIV/AIDS. The maneuver for breaking the impasse was three-pronged: clarity of purpose on the part of the World Bank; emphasis on technical rigor as the basis for any investment in TB and HIV/AIDS control in Russia; and engagement with the highest levels of Russian leadership with concurrent attention to the merit of the case and the importance of face saving.

Regardless of where individual senior officials stood along the spectrum of support for or opposition to WHO-endorsed standards for TB control, there were both overt and covert opposition to using loans from international institutions to finance health in Russia, with the Ministry of Finance leading the pack. With Wieslaw Jakubowiak (WHO's Tuberculosis Program Coordinator in the Russian Federation, based in the Moscow office of WHO) as observer, the World Bank's team presented the Russian delegation with a package of suggestions and options to break the impasse as follows:

- First on the list was to clarify that the World Bank had no interest in selling a loan to Russia if the country did not want it. In fact, the

---

[c] In addition to publicly available publications, this first-hand account is based mostly on (a) the author's recollection from contemporaneous notes and (b) Ref. [20].

message was clear: for the first time, the World Bank was explicitly willing to walk away from loan negotiations, and if Russia wanted the loan, it would need to renew its request for one. We noted that Russia could consider using its own domestic resources for its TB and HIV/AIDS control programs, and the World Bank would be pleased to serve as a partner in program design to the extent that the country wished it to do so alongside other international institutions. I emphasized that the team members' lives would be easier if Russia did not take a loan from the World Bank; the team would diligently engage in strategic, technical, and institutional dimensions of partnering with Russia to tackle TB and HIV/AIDS. The World Bank's main goal was to enable Russia to effectively tackle these challenges and the team would get professional satisfaction from enabling Russia's success in those home-grown objectives without the bureaucratic drudgery of negotiating a loan.

- Second on the list was the emphasis on continuation of technical discussions on a potential Health Reform Implementation Program (HRIP),[22] which was under preparation at the same time. It was a wide-ranging program to support a methodical transformation of the Russian health system from the Soviet inheritance to one that combined quality, efficiency, and relevance to the needs of the population.

  The project would cost $41.21 million, of which the World Bank would finance $30 million. The Russian government would finance the remaining $11.21 million.

  The Government of Canada provided technical assistance to the Chuvash Republic for project preparation through the Canadian International Development Agency (CIDA). The Russian Government's team leader for the HRIP was a highly professional and diligent woman named Nadezhda Lebedeva.

- The third item for consideration was a proposal for a series of Health Policy Seminars to explore opportunities for Russia to lead discussion of its public health and disease control systems and to identify opportunities for their improvement without tying such improvements to any specific financing source. The main activities would include seminars to address selected questions, guided by the following principles:

(i) Russian leadership, including endorsement of the task by policy makers and leadership by Russian experts (as part of this, the process would include adaptation and use of a self-assessment instrument, focusing on the performance of essential public health functions in Russia); (ii) sharing relevant experiences from OECD countries; and (iii) defining options for adoption by the government. During the next two years, Daniel Miller (a senior epidemiologist on secondment from the United States Centers for Disease Control and Prevention to the World Bank) ably co-led with Russian officials the work stream of Public Health Policy Seminars. International participants included some of the best experts in their fields, such as Martin McKee (Professor of European Public Health at the London School of Hygiene and Tropical Medicine), Phyllis Kanki (Professor at the Harvard School of Public Health, who co-discovered HIV-2), and Michael Merson (an internationally recognized expert and leader on HIV/AIDS).

6.4.2 Renewed engagement

A few days after the initial broaching of the three options to resolve the impasse, Russian delegates, led by First Deputy Minister of Health Anatoli Vialkov, stated in Moscow that declining a loan from the World Bank to finance TB and HIV/AIDS control was not a viable option for them. There was pin-drop silence in the room after Mr. Vialkov made this declaration. *Had the Russians been bluffing in public when they declined the loan several months earlier and now reversed positions when their bluff was called in private? Or had they simply rethought their position in the context of a more robust, more flexible, and explicitly less pushy approach by the World Bank?* With no prejudice against their rationale, the dynamics could shift to a combination of rigorous program design, customization for the realities of Russia, coalition building, development of mutually respectful relationships with key Russian entities and international institutions, and strategic communications.

Policy makers in the Russian health sector reached their decision on their own, following careful deliberation. That decision did not primarily derive from conversion to WHO's technical recommendations, but from facing the stark estimates and projections of the potential economic and human damage from unchecked TB and HIV/AIDS. Even those did not come easily. During one memorable session, a senior Russian official dismissed talk about premature deaths from HIV/AIDS, noting that *Mother Russia* lost 25 million to the Great Patriotic War and still thrived, so why should they be overly worried about a few hundreds of thousand potential deaths from HIV/AIDS? Although the rigid opposition to external financing of the TB and HIV/AIDS Control Project was no longer a fundamental problem, there remained potential derailers, which became the focus of consultations and negotiations about the investment in TB and HIV/AIDS control in Russia.

The deeper reason for Russian acceptance of an external loan financing for its TB and HIV/AIDS program derived from a fear of international isolation, dread of further economic devastation, and fear of loss of lives among its working-age population, including its armed forces.

Between October 2001 and June 2002, the World Bank team worked with the Russian Federal AIDS Center to develop estimates and projections of the economic consequences of HIV/AIDS in Russia. The exercise was partly financed by the Department for International Development of the United Kingdom (DFID), with technical support from UNAIDS. Christof Ruehl (the World Bank Economist based in Moscow and lead author of the resulting paper) and I consulted with epidemiologists at UNAIDS (including a session in Geneva in February 2002) to ensure that the epidemiological parameters of the model were robust. Having worked at UNAIDS from 1999 to 2001, I had good contacts there and my former colleagues were both helpful and happy to see the possibility of progress in Russia.

Choosing a forecasting period up until 2020, Ruehl, Pokrovksy, and Vinogradov projected that without any prevention or antiretroviral treatment, the human costs to Russia would be dramatic. They reported the following:[23]

- Even in the optimistic case, mortality rates would increase from 500 per month (2005) to 21,000 per month (2020), and the cumulative number of HIV infected individuals would rise from 1.2 million (2005) to 2.3 (2010) and 5.4 million (2020). The pessimistic scenario resulted in dramatically higher numbers of infections.

- Under similar assumptions, the economic impact on GDP, growth and investment would be substantial: GDP in 2010 would be up to 4.15% lower and without intervention the loss would rise to 10.5% by 2020. Perhaps more significant for long term development, the uninhibited spread of HIV would diminish the economy's long term growth rate, taking off half a percentage point annually by 2010 and a full percentage point annually by 2020.

- *Investment* would decline by more than production. In the pessimistic scenario, its level would decline by 5.5% in 2010 and 14.5% in 2020, indicating more of a stumbling block for future growth.

- Similarly, the *effective*, i.e., quality adjusted *labor supply* would decrease over time. However, a breakdown showed that the overall decline would be due more to a decline in the number of workers ("total labor supply") than to the productivity losses associated with those parts of the work force that would be HIV infected. This reflected the assumption that HIV lowers productivity only by a moderate 13%.

The relationship management and strategic messaging around these findings had a major effect on Russian leaders' attitudes to TB and HIV/ AIDS. Christof Ruehl and I held informal discussions with some senior Russian officials with direct access to the office of the President of the Russian Federation. The understanding was simple and explicit: they would ensure that the information got to the very top, but the World Bank would not pre-emptively disclose that an agreement had been reached. Following that handshake agreement over drinks in a frightfully smoke-filled café in Moscow, they passed the information to their Presidency and pressed for an end to their internal foot-dragging. The bureaucratic and political wheels started to spin faster. In May 2003, President Vladimir Putin mentioned AIDS in a state-of-the-nation speech, a first for a Russian president.

The Economist newspaper, which reported the story in June 2003, provided a colorful rendition of the circumstances.[24] Putin's admission that AIDS was a problem was a triumph of a deliberate strategy by the World Bank team to optimize its engagement for policy decisions based on technical rigor and the investment merit of the case, avoid litigating in the press the sensitive consultations with Russian government officials, and provide Russia with face-saving pathways out of the impasse of 2001. In fact, so successful was this engagement strategy that the study at the core of the Russian turnaround got only a brief mention in the last sentence of *The Economist*'s story, as follows:

> *"So far, AIDS has killed relatively few, a little over 3,000. But unless the government works a lot harder at prevention, that total will swell. A World Bank study predicts that by 2020 up to 10% of an already shrinking population could have the virus — and, long before that, the cost of treating the sick could all but devour the government budget."*

6.4.3 Technical discussions

Providing the Russian government with face-saving pathways also meant a studious avoidance of triumphalism by the World Bank team, key international institutions, and Russian NGOs when Russian government officials changed their positions. This necessitated a functional firewall between two concurrent workstreams. One was the inter-agency Technical Working Group, chaired by the WHO, through which technical parameters were defined, debated, and agreed upon. In addition to major agencies like WHO, the World Bank, USAID (which was engaged in small-scale harm reduction projects), DFID, and UNAIDS, this group also liaised with NGOs, including the Open Society Institute and the Russian Harm Reduction Network. The other workstream was defining an investment program to be financed by a combination of domestic Russian budgets and external financing — principally the World Bank. Details of the former were freely shared. As for the latter, while the World Bank team consulted in technical matters with a number of institutions, and the WHO participated as an observer during negotiations that underpinned the World Bank's investment, specific details of loan negotiations were kept confidential. That approach helped to prevent inadvertent leaks of information that could unwittingly and needlessly anger the Russians, who were very sensitive to perceptions that outsiders might be "helping" them. This

calibration of engagement across multiple parties was noted in an evaluation of the program design process:[25]

> *"In every society in the world in which HIV has been effectively con-*
> *fronted, governments and NGOs have worked in close partnership, most*
> *often with NGOs carrying out programs financed through public*
> *resources. The Russian government, however, retains an impulse to con-*
> *trol third-sector activity (not merely in the HIV arena, but in all areas)*
> *that hinders effective NGO development and program implementation.*
> *The World Bank consulted and collaborated with NGOs in the develop-*
> *ment of the project, particularly in the early stages, but these efforts*
> *have not placed this issue squarely on the government's agenda, in*
> *terms either of government policy toward collaboration with NGOs or*
> *of mechanisms for incorporating NGOs into government sponsored*
> *HIV/AIDS programs. Project documents indicate that a key criterion for*
> *selecting regions for project participation is the availability of HIV-*
> *related NGOs and their capacity for expansion. According to several*
> *NGO-based respondents, however, the project design essentially leaves*
> *the government to determine the degree to which NGOs will be involved*
> *in project implementation."*

Epidemiological and behavioral surveillance of HIV would be done
using methods that were agreed with WHO and UNAIDS.[26] Legislative
barriers to large-scale programs would be eliminated or, at least, reduced.
Science-driven interventions would be key, including the prevention of
HIV infection among IDUs as part of large-scale and targeted interventions among high-risk core transmitters. The program would identify
bridge populations and finance interventions to prevent HIV transmission
in those groups, with a view to preventing transmission from them to the
general population.

The emphasis on epidemiological rigor as a basis for the World
Bank's investment in AIDS control in Russia was markedly different from
that adopted by the Multicountry AIDS Program in the Africa Region of
the World Bank (the Africa MAP), which romanticized populism and
channeling of funds to NGOs. There is nothing inherently wrong about
working with NGOs, as many of them do good work. The problem is that
the MAP's populism came at the expense of a methodical approach to
disease control with grounding in the dynamics of the AIDS epidemic in

Africa; the Africa MAP emphasized populism to the detriment of technical rigor. The independent Operations Evaluation Department of the World Bank found of the Africa MAP that

> "...there is a risk that many of the actors that have been mobilized politically behind the fight against HIV/AIDS are engaged in implementing activities for which they have little capacity, technical expertise, or comparative advantage,"

and that

> "In the absence of strategic advice on prioritization, many of the programs being financed are not sufficiently focused on public goods and reducing high-risk behavior."[27]

6.4.4 Economic analysis

The project appraisal included a project-specific economic analysis of the investment case.[28] Findings from the epidemiological and economic projection models showed that the project would potentially save over 150,000 lives. The benefit:cost ratio was estimated at 7.3. The project would yield a present value of net benefits amounting to US$377 million over five years and about US$1.4 billion over 10 years. Its internal rate of return (IRR) was estimated at 143% (Table 6.1).

Table 6.1.   Summary of Estimated Costs and Benefits

Component	NPV Benefits (US$)		IRR (%)	Benefit: Cost
	5 years	10 years		
AIDS component	16,564,484	172,591,399	77	4.2
TB component	360,583,077	1,205,484,446	215	13.0
Total (both components)	377,147,560	1,378,075,845	143	7.29

NPV benefits is equal to the direct and indirect benefits, minus total project costs. IRR is based on the net benefits over 10 years.

Source: World Bank. 2003. Project Appraisal Document on a Proposed Loan in the Amount of US$150 million to the Russian Federation for a Tuberculosis and AIDS Control Project. Project Appraisal Document. Report Number 21239-RU. http://documents.worldbank.org/en/publication/documents-reports/documentdetail/300501468759013095/Russian-Federation-Tuberculosis-and-AIDS-Control-Project. Accessed on January 7, 2021.

6.4.5 De-escalation and strategic face-saving

One of the priorities of the project was to address local Russian concerns that externally derived DOTS protocols, which WHO approved and which the Word Bank sought to use as the basis for its agreement with Russia, was meant for poor countries and would now be imposed on Russia. Russia would develop its own TB protocols. However, funding from the World Bank would be contingent upon technical agreements between Russia and WHO on the technical integrity of those Russian protocols.[29] In essence, Russia would adopt DOTS and was free to brand it however it wished. This allowed Russian officials to maintain the autonomy of their decision-making while actually accepting international standards. It gave Russian officials who wanted change the cover of a locally viable narrative and the social capital to drive the agenda despite powerful institutional reluctance to change. The protocols would be specific to Russia while keeping international guidelines at their core.

Another important item during negotiations was an explicit clarification that Russia would not use the World Bank loan to purchase technical support from WHO. WHO would finance its own work from other sources. This resolved a major source of concerns for the Russian Ministry of Finance while keeping WHO at the technical core of the work. In addition, it provided a reference for politely — and firmly — declining informal requests from a couple of Western NGOs for their staff salaries to be paid from the proceeds of the World Bank loan.

The procurement of second-line drugs for treating TB was another major issue. The solution lay in finding methods that would be acceptable to the Russian Government and the World Bank. Eligible methods included but crucially were not limited to International Competitive Bidding (ICB). During the earlier phases of discussion of the program, powerful stakeholders in Russia (especially Russia-based pharmaceutical companies) had opposed the potential loan. They feared that the importation of quality-assured and inexpensive second-line medicines for MDR-TB would be bad for their own businesses. The parties agreed that the use of loan proceeds to purchase second-line medicines for treating MDR-TB would be contingent upon WHO verification of their compliance with technical guidelines on quality assurance. The World Bank agreed to explore sources that could support the local industry with a view to enabling them to attain Good Manufacturing Practice (GMP) standards. The World Bank also facilitated the early stage of a potential transfer of technology from pharmaceutical companies that produced second-line anti-TB medicines to eligible Russian enterprises.

Lastly, it must be noted that despite some journalists' feverish interest in the case, the World Bank team did not disclose to them any information on specifics of the negotiations. However, even after the Russian Government and the World Bank signed off on the formal negotiations, one journalist reported that there were no conditions on procurement.[30] By then, it did not matter; sometimes, radio silence is the best communication.

6.5. Resolution

In routine situations, negotiations of investment loan agreements such as that in Russia tend to be low-key affairs led by lawyers. This is because any contentious issue of strategy or technical design would have been resolved during the earlier stages of work, which included project preparation, pre-appraisal, and appraisal. But the engagement in Russia was far from routine. The Russian Ministry of Finance was stalling on naming its delegation to formally negotiate the loan with the World Bank in Moscow. Those negotiations were scheduled to start on Monday, December 16, 2002 and be concluded on Friday, December 20, 2002. The informal word in Moscow was that Alexander Pavlov, the MOF's Deputy Head of the International Cooperation and External Debt Management Department, for unspecified reasons, still opposed the loan investment. In such situations, the World Bank's project team would normally not depart from Washington DC for the purpose of Negotiations. However, given that the overt obstacles to an agreement had been eliminated and that the topmost echelons of the Russian Government favored the investment, I decided in agreement with Schweitzer (World Bank Country Director for Russia) to travel from Washington DC to Moscow for a Technical Discussion with the Russian counterparts. The records of a Technical Discussion, if successful, could be upgraded to Agreed Negotiations via an exchange of signatures later.

Once the Washington-based members of the World Bank team arrived in Moscow, word spread across the Moscow-based international agencies and Russian government officials working on the proposed project that matters were coming to a head. It was time for the Russian Ministry of Finance to finally fish or cut bait on the potential loan investment in TB and AIDS Control. We had a superb team, some of whom were in Moscow during that period. Maria Gracheva (the pin-sharp, no-nonsense World Bank Operations Officer) combined with Paolo Giribona (biomedical engineer and consultant to the World Bank on medical equipment) to clarify any issues that remained in procurement and operations management. Tatyana Loginova, with an encyclopedic knowledge of key Russian actors and interests, untangled the political signals from the noise across ministries and institutions. Wieslaw Jakubowiak of the WHO was an able broker at the interface between WHO and the World Bank.

There was just one problem: initially, no senior Russian official showed up, even for Technical Discussions, in the Moscow office of the World Bank. Then they started trickling in until there was a quorum for robust discussions. At this point, Schweitzer and I executed a pre-agreed gambit. Julian Schweitzer walked into the meeting room, effusively thanked all those in attendance for their hard work, and promptly announced that although he had agreed to host these Technical Discussions in recognition of its importance to Russia, the World Bank team had just about exhausted its administrative budget for preparing the TB and AIDS Control Project in Russia. Therefore, he stressed, if Negotiations were not concluded during this round of talks, he would have no objection to the team coming back to Moscow, but there would be no additional World Bank administrative budget for such work and I, as the Team Leader, would have to find the money from my own pocket.

That tactic worked. Despite much haggling over some details, the Technical Discussions progressed. But it wasn't over. At one point, a couple of Russian officials again queried the rationale for tackling MDR-TB. I had deliberately worn a TB necktie in anticipation of precisely such stalling tactics. I stood up, turned the necktie inside out, and read the following text inscribed on the tie from *Infectious Awareables*, on which were colorful artworks of the tubercle bacillus and infected cells:

"Tuberculosis is a chronic bacterial infection, usually affecting the lungs, transmitted by inhalation of infected airborne droplets. Adherence to treatment regimen is critical in order to reduce incidence of multiple drug resistance."

Participants, including the Russian delegation, burst into laughter. The pointlessness of querying the rationale for tackling MDR-TB *at that late stage* was clear to all. The tension in the room evaporated. Importantly, nobody lost face. The Technical Discussions continued until they were agreed upon and signed by the Russian government and the World Bank delegates on December 20, 2002.

But the real need was for those Agreed Minutes of Technical Discussions to be upgraded to Agreed Minutes of Negotiations. The mid-ranking officer from the Ministry of Finance, a highly professional woman named Natalia V. Polukarova (Deputy Head of Unit, International Cooperation and External Debt Management Department, MOF) was not officially authorized to participate in the discussions because of opposition by her boss Alexander Pavlov. But she showed up anyway and later explained that she had done so out of a sense of duty and her observation that the World Bank team truly understood and wanted to assist Russia in tackling its health problems. Then the Minister of Finance, who had been traveling outside Russia, returned to Moscow just before the weekend, and word got to him about the stumbling block. The MOF dynamics changed during informal back-and-forth that weekend.

By the evening of Sunday, December 22, 2002, it seemed that the last hurdle was resolved and likely that we would complete Negotiations on the next day. But likelihood is not the same as certainty, and I was concerned that a loss of momentum at that stage could again derail the program. Just in case the talks dragged on, I called home to alert my family that I might not be home in time for Christmas.

The Agreed Minutes of Negotiations were signed on Monday, December 23, 2002 in the Russian Ministry of Health in Moscow. The agreement paved the way for the Board of Directors of the World Bank to formally approve the agreement with Russia for the $286 million Tuberculosis and AIDS Control Project, of which the World Bank loan would finance US$150 million. That approval would come later on April 3, 2003.

The Russian delegation to the December 23, 2002 session included senior officials from the Ministry of Health, Ministry of Justice, and Ministry of Finance, representing a broader group that included the Ministry of Economic Development and Trade, and the Ministry of Industry, Science and Technology. The World Bank delegation noted that upon signing, the Negotiations would be finished, and the next steps would be largely procedural, paving the way for implementation.

Just after the Russian and World Bank officials signed the papers, several Russian cameramen, including one holding a video camera, entered the room. As if on cue, the Russian Health Minister Yuri L. Shevchenko, who led the Russian delegation to the Negotiations, looked at the cameras, then, turning to Schweitzer and me, proclaimed:

"We all know that our experts are better than yours."

In the bitterly cold early morning of December 24, 2002, Mr. Boris, a diligent driver of his own taxi, drove me from the hotel across the road from the Red Square to the Sheremetyevo airport. Few sights are as stunning as the Red Square after heavy snowfall, when those famous domes seem otherworldly. Boris drove slowly so that I could take in the sight one more time. The ashes of Yuri Gagarin, the first human to travel into outer space, are buried in the Kremlin Wall Necropolis. Decades earlier, I had small posters of Gagarin and Neil Armstrong on a locker in my high school. Boris had an encyclopedic knowledge of Russian operas and had given me an overview of "Boris Godunov" before I saw it at the Bolshoi Theater. He had figured that I liked Louis Armstrong's "What A Wonderful World." We would hum along as he played it in his old but clean and reliable Volvo. We might not win a Grammy, but the spirit was always good. As we approached the airport, I suggested that we sing something different and he obliged. He smiled when he realized what I was struggling to hum, and with gusto, we jointly belted out *Kalinka*.

References

[1] Erofeyev Y. 2002. The Russian God. *The New Yorker*. https://www.newyorker.com/magazine/2002/12/16/the-russian-god. Accessed on April 11, 2021.

[2] U.S. Department of State. A Guide to the United States' History of Recognition, Diplomatic, and Consular Relations, by Country, since 1776: Russia. https://history.state.gov/countries/russia. Accessed on December 22, 2020.

[3] Barr N. 1994. From transition to accession. In *Labor Markets and Social Policy in Central and Eastern Europe*. The World Bank. pp. 3–10. https://elibrary.worldbank.org/doi/abs/10.1596/0-8213-6119-8.

[4] Yablonksii P, Vizel A, Galkin V, Shulgina M. 2015. Tuberculosis in Russia. Its history and its status today. *American Journal of Respiratory and Critical Care Medicine*. https://www.atsjournals.org/doi/full/10.1164/rccm.201305-0926OE.

[5] World Health Organization. Global tuberculosis control: WHO report 2011, WHO/HTM/TB/2011.16. http://whqlibdoc.who.int/publications/2011/9789241564380_eng.pdf. Accessed on January 8, 2021.

[6] Reichman LB. 2002. Timebomb: The Global Epidemic of Multi-drug Resistant Tuberculosis, pp. 63–126. McGraw-Hill.

[7] Dyce C, Williams B, Espinal MA, Raviglione M. 2002. Erasing the world's slow stain: Strategies to beat multidrug-resistant Tuberculosis. *Science, 295*: 2042–2046.

[8] Espinal MA, Kim SJ, Suarez PG, Kam KM, Khomenko AG, Migliori GB, *et al.* 2000. Standard short-course chemotherapy for drug-resistant Tuberculosis: Treatment outcomes in 6 countries. *JAMA,* 283(19): 2537–2545.

[9] Bennetts M. 2020. The epidemic Russia doesn't want to talk about. https://www.politico.eu/article/everything-you-wanted-to-know-about-aids-in-russia-but-putin-was-afraid-to-ask/. Accessed on December 30, 2020.

[10] UNAIDS and WHO. 2002. AIDS Epidemic Update. https://www.who.int/hiv/pub/epidemiology/epi2002/en/#:~:text=Summary,million%20of%20them%20were%20women. Accessed on January 9, 2021.

[11] Rhodes T, Lowndes C, Judd A, *et al.* 2002. Explosive spread and high prevalence of HIV infection among injecting drug users in Togliatti City, Russia. *AIDS,* Sep 6, 16(13): F25–31. doi: 10.1097/00002030-200209060-00002.

[12] Eaton W J. 1989. Soviets Hail Andrei Gromyko, Dead at 79, as 'Devoted Soldier'. https://www.latimes.com/archives/la-xpm-1989-07-04-mn-3333-story.html. Accessed on December 30, 2020.

[13] Mallaby S. 2004. *The World's Banker. A Story of Failed States, Financial Crises, and the Wealth and Poverty of Nations*. The Penguin Press: New York, pp. 313–335.

[14] Glasser SB. 2001. Russia Balks at World Bank TB Aid. *The Washington Post*, May 8, 2001. https://www.washingtonpost.com/archive/politics/2001/05/08/russia-balks-at-world-bank-tb-aid/3cbbe53a-17db-490a-b273-b472e55b83cf/. Accessed on December 29, 2020.

[15] WHO. 2002. *Global Tuberculosis Control: Surveillance, Planning, Financing.* Geneva: World Health Organization.

[16] Hamers F, Downs A. 2003. HIV in central and eastern Europe. *The Lancet*, 361: 1035–1044.

[17] WHO and UNAIDS. 2000. Guidelines for Second Generation Surveillance. WHO/CDS/CSR/ECD/2000.5, UNAIDS/00.03E. Geneva.

[18] Schwartlander B, Gys P, Pisani E, Kiesssling S, Lazzari S, Carael M, *et al.* 2001. HIV surveillance in hard-to-reach populations. *AIDS*, 15(suppl 3): S1–S3

[19] Heifets L. 2003. WHO and Russia: The turning point in joint efforts against TB. *International Journal of Tuberculosis and Lund Disease*, 7(2): 1–2

[20] Adeyi O, Fidler A, Gracheva M, Loginova T. 2003/2004. Tuberculosis and AIDS control in Russia: Closing the knowing-doing gap. *Eurohealth*, 9(4)Winter: 22–277. https://www.lse.ac.uk/lse-health/assets/documents/eurohealth/issues/eurohealth-v9n4.pdf. Accessed on June 18, 2021.

[21] McPherson JM. 2007. *This Mighty Scourge: Perspectives on the Civil War.* Oxford University Press: New York, pp. 93–108.

[22] World Bank. Health Reform Implementation Project. Information Page. https://projects.worldbank.org/en/projects-operations/document-detail/P046497. Accessed on January 13, 2021.

[23] Ruehl C, Pokrovksy V, Vinogradov V. 2002. The Economic Consequences of HIV in Russia. May 2002. This report is no longer on the website of the World Bank Country Office for Russia.

[24] AIDS in Russia: Saying Versus Doing. June 2003. https://www.economist.com/europe/2003/06/19/saying-versus-doing.

[25] Twigg J, Skolnik R. 2005. Evaluation of the World Bank's Assistance in Responding to the AIDS Epidemic: Russia Case Study. *The World Bank Operations Evaluation Department*, pp. 35–36. https://www.semanticscholar.org/paper/Evaluation-of-the-World-Bank%E2%80%99s-Assistance-in-to-the-Twigg-Skolnik/41b0971126d0d4a0f303757965dfa636f6845801. Accessed on January 7, 2021.

[26] Dehne C, Pokrosvksy V, Kobyscha Y, Schwartlander B. 2000. Update on the epidemics of HIV and other sexually transmitted infections in the new independent states of the former Soviet Union. *AIDS*, 14(suppl 3):S75–S84.

[27] Operations Evaluation Department. 2005. Committing to Results: Improving the Effectiveness of HIV/AIDS Assistance, An OED Evaluation of the World Bank's Assistance for HIV/AIDS Control. Washington, DC: World Bank. © World Bank. https://openknowledge.worldbank.org/handle/10986/7435 License: CC BY 3.0 IGO. https://openknowledge.worldbank.org/handle/10986/7435. Accessed on January 11, 2021.

[28] World Bank. 2003. Project Appraisal Document on a Proposed Loan in the Amount of US$150 million to the Russian Federation for a Tuberculosis and AIDS Control Project. Project Appraisal Document. Report Number 21239-RU. http://documents.worldbank.org/en/publication/documents-reports/document detail/300501468759013095/Russian-Federation-Tuberculosis-and-AIDS-Control-Project. Accessed on January 7, 2021.

[29] Heifets L. 2003. WHO and Russia: The turning point in joint efforts against TB. *International Journal of Tuberculosis and Lung Disease*, 7(2):1–2. https://www.ingentaconnect.com/contentone/iuatld/ijtld/2003/00000007/00000002/art00001#. Accessed on April 22, 2021.

[30] Webster P. 2002. Agreement unlocks loan for TB and AIDS treatment in Russia. *Science,* Jul 12, 297(5579): 170. DOI: 10.1126/science.297.5579.170. https://science.sciencemag.org/content/297/5579/170.full. Accessed on January 7, 2021.

Chapter 7

Health System in Nigeria: Investors' Dream or Nightmare?

"Here in Nigeria, people seem to accept the unacceptable revelations of how politicians share millions of Naira belonging to the nation. The newspapers report them and the television speaks about them, but people just laugh; they laugh because they have been shocked to the state of unshockability."

—Dele Giwa[a]

Synopsis

This chapter examines the Nigerian health system through the lenses of political history, contemporary policy goals, financing, health status, domestic political economy, and the engagement between Nigeria-based experts and their external counterparts. Fundamental to this chapter is that wallowing in the past is not the solution to current challenges. Doing so would absolve recent and current policy makers of responsibility, and it would infantilize and deny the agency of the population. However, understanding the past helps to explain much of the present and provides a basis to enable a better future.

---

[a]Giwa D. 1986. Nobody cares. *Newswatch.* https://www.thecable.ng/nobody-cares-dele-giwa. Accessed on February 22, 2021.

Four interlinked issues are of interest: the realities of Nigeria's quest for Universal Health Coverage (UHC) via a viable health system; financing of the health system and the dynamics at play during legislation, budgeting, and implementation; the realities of Development Assistance for Health (DAH); and opportunities for better performance. The chapter combines data with attention to the functions of institutions and the compact — or lack of same — between the government and the governed in matters of health.

7.1. Lugard's Tropical Alchemy

Nigeria was created by fiat on January 1, 1914. Michael Crowder, in *The Story of Nigeria*,[1] narrates the geopolitics, contemporary forces, and expediencies that explained the internal logic of the decision made by Sir Frederick Lugard, the luxuriantly mustachioed British Governor-General, to amalgamate the Northern Protectorate and the Southern Protectorate of Nigeria. Within Britain's fundamentally economic and exploitative interest in Nigeria, the logic was impeccable:

> *"The immediate reason for the decision to amalgamate the two Nigerias was economic expediency. The Northern Protectorate was running at a severe deficit, which was being met by a subsidy from the Southern Protectorate, and an Imperial Grant-in-Aid from Britain of about £300,000 a year. This conflicted with the age-old colonial policy that each territory should be self-sustaining. Apart from the fact that it seemed logical to amalgamate the two territories, the one land-locked and the other with a long seaboard, it was felt that the prosperous Southern Protectorate could subsidize its northern neighbor until such time as it became self-supporting.*
>
> *By centralizing the Treasury, Lugard was able to divert revenue that earlier had been properly the South's to balance the Northern deficit."*

Modern-day barons of DAH might recognize, perhaps with envy, the brilliance of Lugard's move — from the colonizer's perspective. In one stroke, he relieved Westminster of the potential burden of subsidizing a foreign entity and created a notionally sustainable colony. Lugard's ingenuity in the service of his sovereign was recognized during his own lifetime. He retired in 1919 to life as a guru on colonialism and held the title of Baron Lugard of Abinger. With his expertise on *the natives*, he served as chair of the International Institute of African Languages and Cultures, and was a member of the International Committees on Slavery and Forced Labor. He authored a book, *Dual Mandate in British Tropical Africa,* which was published in 1922.[2]

The priors of amalgamation in Nigeria are familiar to those with more than a cursory knowledge of the history of Africa. There were intersocietal commerce, socialization, and wars. There was the singularly crippling torture, capture, and sale of Africans as slaves across the Atlantic. The facts of how Europe crushed, subjugated, and underdeveloped Africa in pursuit of its own economic self-interest are well documented.[3–7] Belgium's extraordinary crimes against humanity in the Congo[8] receive colorful portrayals, but the Belgians did not have a monopoly of using force through punitive expeditions to, in their framing, teach sense to the *natives*[9] while falsely casting indigenous African empires as primitive people to be civilized. Britain was just as guilty.[10] These actions set the stage for colonialism and they frame the post-colonial evolution of Nigeria and its health system. A seed of inequity of access came early, as access to the first generation of colonial health facilities was initially for Europeans only. Out of commercial self-interest, it was later extended to Africans who worked for European establishments.[11]

7.2. Six Decades of Policies and Implementation after Independence

In the six decades since independence, Nigeria has enacted multiple policy positions and policies on health. While some were domestic in origin and inspiration, others were in response to global pronouncements and movements in the form of Primary Health Care (PHC)[12] and UHC.[13]

The period from 1960 to 1980 started with little attention to health systems, with emphasis mostly on the infrastructure for curative care.[14,15] From 1975 to 1980, health system development received attention, with emphasis on PHC,[16] and the advent of the National Basic Health Services Scheme (NBHSS). Professor Olikoye Ransome-Kuti led the adoption of PHC, first in a pilot phase and then across the entire country. He also ensured the development of Nigeria's first comprehensive National Health Policy, which was grounded in PHC and launched in 1988.[17] Professor Adetokunbo Lucas, who chaired the Committee on National Health Policy that was convened in 1984, recalled the events as follows:[18]

> *"Our report was brief and to the point. We recommended that the governments of Nigeria should adopt Primary Health Care (PHC) as the key to health development in the nation. The report set out the main features of a health system based on PHC. It provided a skeletal framework that would be developed in operational terms.*
>
> *The presentation of our report was attended by the usual fanfare with wide media coverage. In presenting the document, I noted that similar reports had been abandoned on the shelf to collect dust; nothing was done to implement the recommendations. I urged the government to review our report and implement the proposed strategies. The Minister thanked members of the committee and there followed a ray of hope as I was invited to present our report to the National Council on Health, the body that coordinates health among the states of the Federation. It turned out to be a full stop for neither the Minister of Health nor the two ministers who succeeded him took action to implement the national health policy. The breakthrough came with the appointment of Professor Olikoye Ransome-Kuti as the Minister of Health. Within days of taking power, General Babangida recalled Ransome-Kuti's lecture at the ministry Staff College proposing PHC as the best basis for the Nigerian health system. General Babangida asked him to implement these ideas that he presented at the lecture. I drew the attention of the new minister to our report that had been gathering dust on the shelf. Through his determined effort, the National Executive Council accepted the report and endorsed the new policy. Professor Ransome-Kuti then studiously set in motion reforms of the health system to as to develop PHC. Before leaving office, he created the National Primary Health Care Development Agency (NPHCDA) as a parastatal organization with responsibility for promoting and supporting PHC. Thus, he earned the title of being the father of Nigerian primary health care."*

The progress and challenges under the PHC initiative are well covered elsewhere in the literature.[19–22] In a cross-cutting study, Kress and others reported on the multiple dimensions of systemic underperformance in Nigeria's health system. They emphasized "two overarching system-level challenges — financing and governance — that are key root causes of the dysfunctions observed in the PHC system in Nigeria."[23]

7.3. Poor Health Outcomes Undermining Human Capital

"I have never regarded myself as having a monopoly of wisdom. The trouble is that when most people in life and in the position of leadership and rulership are spending whole days and nights carousing in clubs or in the company of men of shady character and women of easy virtue, I, like a few others, am always at my post working hard at the country's problems, and trying to find solutions for them. Only the deep can call to the deep. This is the difference."

—Obafemi Awolowo

By the most commonly used measures of the most basic aggregate health outcomes, Nigeria's current health status is poor compared to most plausible comparators (Table 7.1). The country fares worse than the Africa-wide benchmarks for healthy life expectancy at birth, maternal mortality ratio, and under-five mortality rate (U5MR).

Nigeria's U5MR is both high and inequitable across income groups. For children in the poorest income quintile, Nigeria has the highest U5MR in West Africa. Within the country, children from the poorest quintile die at a rate that is 3.3 times higher than for those from the richest quintile. Population coverage of *high-quality* essential health services is poor.[24]

The countrywide aggregate outcomes mask important variations across zones and states within the country. These disparities have multiple causes, both historical and contemporary. The variations across geopolitical zones and states are large. Indicators such as those for maternal and child health service coverage and outcomes correlate with educational status and wealth.[25] Given these findings of poor outcomes at the country level and major disparities in performance within the country, an investor

Table 7.1.   **Health Outcomes and Service Coverage: Nigeria in the Global Context**

WHO Region/ Country	Healthy Life Expectancy at Birth (years)	Maternal Mortality Ratio. MMR. (per 100,000 live births)	Under 5 Mortality Rate. U5MR. (per 1,000 live births)	UHC Service Coverage Index	Population (%) with Household Expenditures >10% of Total Household Expenditure or Income	Average of 13 International Health Regulations Core Capacity Scores
	2016	2017	2018	2017	2010–2018	2019
Africa	53.8	525	76	46	7.3	44
The Americas	67.5	57	14	79	11.3	71
South-East Asia	60.4	152	34	56	16.0	61
Europe	68.4	13	9	77	7.4	75
Eastern Mediterranean	59.7	164	47	57	11.7	66
Western Pacific	68.9	41	12	77	15.9	71
Global	63.3	211	39	66	12.7	63
Nigeria	48.9	917	120	42	15.1	51

Source: Adapted from WHO. World Health Statistics 2020. https://www.who.int/data/gho/publications/world-health-statistics. Accessed on February 16, 2021.

who is optimizing for improved health outcomes would, all other things being equal, aim to achieve improved overall performance *and* equity through a combination of improvements in every state *and* comparatively more rapid improvements in the lagging parts of the country. That quest makes sense and is especially important in the context of another driver of health outcomes: education.

There are significant positive associations between education and the use of maternal health services in Nigeria.[26] The wide variations in literacy rates have roots in cross-regional variations in education policies and school enrollment.[27] In the mid-1950s, the Government of the Western Region, led by the late Obafemi Awolowo, initiated a policy of Universal Free Primary Education. The Eastern Region soon took similar steps. The Northern Region was a relative laggard in this regard and has not taken the same vigorous and relentless approach as the other regions. More specifically, as reported by Adetoro in 1966:[28]

"Since 1955, when the Western Region Government triggered off the education race by the introduction of a Universal Free Primary Education Scheme, there has been a remarkable growth, at least quantitatively, in nearly all sectors of Nigerian education. The most substantial growth has, of course, been recorded at the primary school level. As an illustration, there was a countrywide enrolment of only 560,000 pupils in the primary schools in 1946. In 1954, the Western Region alone enrolled 340,610 boys and 115,990 girls — a total of 455,700 in 4,373 primary schools. The government envisaged that some 150,000 children in the 6–7 age group would be registered in the first year of the free primary school scheme which was due to start the following year. This proved to be a great underestimation as in fact, 391,891 Class I pupils became the first beneficiaries of free schooling. The total primary school population during the first year of the scheme was 811,432. By 1958, enrolment had passed the one million mark. In 1963, the year for which the latest statistics are available, there were 1,099,418 pupils in 6,311 primary schools in the Western Region.

The statistics for Eastern Nigeria are equally impressive. In 1952, there were in the region 3,521 primary schools with a combined enrolment of 518,948. During 1957 — the first year of that region's own scheme of free primary education — the schools had multiplied to 6,654 and there were 1,194,354 children attending them. The Lagos primary education scheme also started in 1957 with 50,182 pupils in 96 schools. In 1962, the number of Lagos schools had increased to 120 and enrolment was 90,511. Even in the Northern Region, which has not yet embarked upon its free primary education project, a three-fold increase was recorded in school population between 1948 and 1958."

Two generations later, the effects of those divergent policies are playing out in 21st-century Nigeria, as indicated in Table 7.2.

Figure 7.1 shows the large variations in the Total Fertility Rate (TFR) across states in Nigeria.

The combination of underperformance in health and education shows in the Human Capital Index: among all countries in the Human Capital Index, Nigeria ranked 7th from the bottom, ahead of only Liberia, Mali,

Table 7.2.   Inequality and Education of Women in Nigeria

Zone of Nigeria	Gini Coefficient	Women Aged 15–49 Years with No Formal Education (%)	Women Aged 15–49 Years with Higher than Secondary Schooling (%)	Women Aged 15–49 Years Who Are Literate (%)
North Central	0.27	31.8	10.7	49.6
North East	0.33	59.1	6.2	31.8
North West	0.33	63.8	4.5	29.0
South East	0.17	4.2	15.4	79.3
South South	0.16	4.7	15.7	79.0
South West	0.13	7.9	20.4	80.6

Source: Adapted from Nigeria Demographic and Health Survey 2018. https://www.dhsprogram.com/publications/publication-fr359-dhs-final-reports.cfm. Accessed on February 17, 2021.

Niger, South Sudan, Chad, and the Central African Republic.[29] In a world that is increasingly driven and dominated by knowledge economies, such abysmally low performance in human capital does not bode well for growth and competitiveness. The challenge is more basic than competing with other countries in a knowledge-driven 21st Century. It is also not for a lack of exceptionally accomplished Nigerians. There are Nigerians who excel in just about every field of endeavor. But there is a difference between individual brilliance and collective effectiveness as a country. The superbly accomplished and motivated Nigerians show how far the country *can* go. However, it is the tens of millions of uneducated and unskilled people who will determine how far the country *will* go. On that basis, Nigeria *as a country* has not decisively committed to the global race to the top.

7.4. Service Delivery and Systemic Dysfunctions

Data on the most basic and predictable health services show low coverage levels (even without accounting for quality of care) and wide variations across zones and states. The two indicators of service delivery used for illustration here are delivery in a health facility and childhood vaccination. They were chosen because the need for these basic services is foreseeable

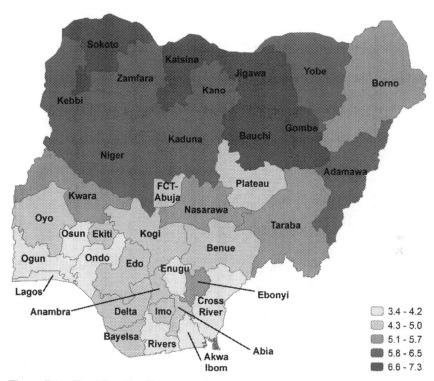

Figure 7.1.   Total Fertility Rate by State

Source: Nigeria Demographic and Health Survey. 2018. https://www.dhsprogram.com/publications/ publication-fr359-dhs-final-reports.cfm. Accessed on February 17, 2021.

and thus largely amenable to effective planning, demand generation, and assurance of supply. Figure 7.2 shows dramatic interstate variations in the percentage of live births in the 5 years before the survey that were delivered in a health facility.

Vaccination coverage in Nigeria improved in the decade leading to the last Demographic and Health (DHS) survey of 2018. However, the starting point was a low base and the status at the time of the survey was still poor. Figure 7.3 shows by state the percentage of children aged 12–23 months who received all basic vaccines at any time before the survey.

It has been noted that access to the health system's physical infrastructure is not the binding constraint on the effective coverage of PHC in Nigeria. More than 80% of the population live within 30-minute travel of a health facility. The systemic underperformance is rooted in a

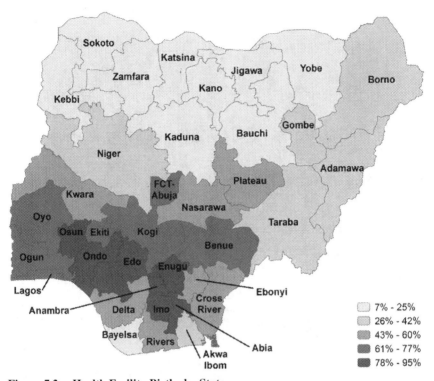

Figure 7.2. Health Facility Births by State

Source: Nigeria Demographic and Health Survey. 2018. https://www.dhsprogram.com/publications/publication-fr359-dhs-final-reports.cfm. Accessed on February 17, 2021.

combination of weak health system management, financial barriers to access, poor knowledge that constrains care-seeking behavior, limited mobility, poorly incentivized and supervised health workers, inadequate accountability, and gender norms.[24]

Multiple factors drive the underperformance of the health system in Nigeria.[25] In matters of health, there is no compact between the government and the population of the sort that would have electoral consequences for poor performance by politicians. This context is devoid of mutual accountabilities among principals, agents, and citizens,[30] and it does not work for the poor. The reasons include entrenched rent seeking, patronage, corruption,[31] and the disdain with which the elite appear to treat the masses.[32,33] Weak public financial management enables

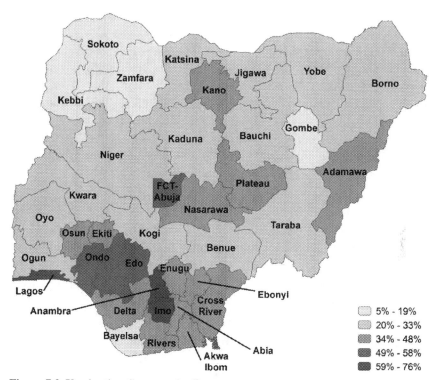

Figure 7.3. Vaccination Coverage by State

Source: Nigeria Demographic and Health Survey 2018. https://www.dhsprogram.com/publications/publication-fr359-dhs-final-reports.cfm. Accessed on February 17, 2021.

mismanagement and corruption. Smith's conclusions on Nigeria's anti-corruption efforts merit a close look:[34]

> *"Over and above the technocratic features of particular policies, programs, and related efforts to curtail corruption in Nigeria, two main — and often intertwining — aspects of the problem are at the core of whether anticorruption initiatives in Nigeria will succeed or fail. The first is the problem of political elites.[35] The second is ordinary citizens and their role in reproducing a culture of corruption as it contradicts their ultimate interests.[36] With regard to elites, Lawson notes in her analysis of the politics of anticorruption in Africa more generally, "those called upon to make the structural changes to limit opportunities for corruption are the very actors who benefit most from the status*

quo."[37] In Nigeria, as elsewhere, anticorruption campaigns pose a serious danger to the material interests of elites.[38] Corruption, many have argued, is part of the very fabric of power in Nigeria, a defining element of the state[36,37,39] As such, rooting it out requires more than just formal anticorruption policies and programs.

The challenges to effective anticorruption efforts are exacerbated by the fact that even ordinary Nigerians have become invested in certain practices of corruption ... while Nigerians are generally socially supportive of anti-corruption efforts, many are politically and economically connected to the corruption complex, directly or indirectly."[38]

This is not to imply that corruption is uniquely Nigerian. A couple of examples will suffice to debunk any such notion. Washington DC, the capital of the United States, has a street where lobbyists tend to set up shop. K Street, in the North-West quadrant of the city, is the place to be for professional peddlers and purchasers of influence which, in plainspeak, is codified corruption in plain sight. Readers who seek a primer in this remarkable American approach are encouraged to read *This Town*.[40] Despite pledges to drain the swamp in the 2016 United States election campaigns, it appeared that not only did the alligators of K Street increase in number during the next four years, but they grew on steroids. Across the Atlantic, the question is addressed in the aptly titled *How Corrupt is Britain?*[41] Former UK Prime Minister David Cameron, of whom it is written that his "political afterlife reveals a zone where accountability dissolves,"[42] reportedly asserted that Nigeria is "fantastically corrupt."[43,44] His assertion has merit; Nigeria has advanced beyond the kind of murkiness in which Mr. Cameron is reportedly enmeshed[45,46] and surpassed its former colonial overlords at their own game. That is no mean feat, given London's centrality to corruption as eloquently noted in a *Guardian* newspaper editorial in 2016:[47]

"The prime minister is not personally corrupt — but he is certainly guilty of epic hypocrisy. So, for that matter, are Britain and the west. They have spent decades ordering poor countries and failed states to sort out their problems with dodgy money, even while taking much of that dodgy money and ploughing it through their banks, their ritzy

stores, their estate agents, and their offshore tax havens — with barely any questions asked or eyebrows raised. When Mr Cameron was caught on camera on Tuesday boasting to the Queen of the "fantastically corrupt countries" turning up at Lancaster House this week, he might have mentioned that Afghanistan is a failed state that did not get any less failed over 13 years of British intervention. And he should certainly have mentioned that the president of Nigeria, Muhammadu Buhari, is coming to London to lobby it to sort out the tax havens in its own backyard. Indeed, Mr Cameron might have quoted a letter sent to him a fortnight ago by campaigners in Nigeria.

"We are embarked on a nationwide anti-corruption campaign," the letter said. "But these efforts are sadly undermined if countries such as your own are welcoming our corrupt to hide their ill-gotten gains in your luxury homes, department stores, car dealerships, private schools and anywhere else that will accept their cash with no questions asked. The role of London's property market as vessels to conceal stolen wealth has been exposed in court documents, reports, documentaries and more." So the president of the Nigerian senate, Bukola Saraki, currently facing allegations that he failed to declare his assets, owns a property in London's Belgravia in his own name. But last month's Panama Papers revealed that the £5.7m property next door is owned by companies incorporated in the Seychelles and British Virgin Islands, whose respective shareholders are Saraki's wife and former special assistant. And a £1.65m townhouse in Kensington is shown as belonging to a BVI company whose sole shareholder is Folorunsho Coker, former head of the number plate production authority of the state of Lagos and currently business adviser to the governor of Lagos. None of these individuals may have done anything wrong, but the charge from those campaigners is hard to duck. Under successive governments, from Thatcher to Blair to Cameron, London has become the financial center for the world's dirty money."

There is debate about whether rooting out corruption is a necessary precondition for development, or whether anticorruption efforts gain traction as a result of economic development.[48] Regardless of the direction of causality over time in that debate, both domestic (including public) and foreign (including DAH)[49,50] investments take on higher risks when corruption drains funds from their intended purpose. Onwujekwe and colleagues note the complexity of systemic corruption and the difficulty of identifying and tackling corruption in situations where there is opacity in the rules or where enforcement is lax.[51] The ultimate point is that corruption in Nigeria impedes systemic performance and health outcomes, with disproportionate effects on the less privileged.[52]

The reality is that while there are thousands of health workers who strive to perform their duties, systemic failures have prevented the achievement of effective coverage of the population with health services. The publicly funded hospitals at State and Federal levels are reputed to have poor quality of care. The system lacks an integration of evidence-based planning, research, and statistics to inform policies, enable rational resource allocation choices, and make explicit the performance of the health system at all levels.[53,54]

7.5. Financing: Positive Signs and Perils

An overview of government structure and legislation helps to understand the promise and perils of health financing in Nigeria. The design of the Federal system — which provides concurrent responsibilities for the Local, State, and Federal Governments — has features that complicate policy formulation and the coordination for implementation across the three levels.[55,56] The structure of fiscal federalism, that is, the allocation of tax authority, revenue mobilization, and expenditure responsibilities across the three levels of government, adds complexity to governance. It is possible that increasing subnational autonomy could enhance representative governance and accountability,[57] but that is not guaranteed because of a mismatch between the capabilities of the Local Governments (which have prime responsibility for delivering PHC services) and the level of organizational and managerial skills required to effectively perform those functions.

Evolutions in policy and legislation have led to the National Health Act of 2014.[58] By design, it was potentially very consequential. The intentions met reality at the point of translation from law to budgets and the translation of policy into practice. A starting point for unpacking the issues and identifying opportunities for improvement is the summary of health financing in Nigeria, shown in the global context in Table 7.3. It

Table 7.3. Health Financing in Nigeria in the Global Context

Country Group/Specific Country	Health Spending per Capita, 2016 (US$)	Health Spending per Capita, 2016 ($PPP)	Health Spending per GDP, 2016 (%)	Government Health Spending per Total Health Spending, 2016	Out of Pocket Spending per Total Health Spending (%)	DAH per Total Health Spending, 2016 (%)
High income	5,252	5,621	10.8	79.6	13.8	0
Upper-middle income	491	1,009	5.0	53.9	53.9	0.2
Lower-middle income	81	274	3.2	32.1	56.1	3.2
Low income	40	125	5.1	26.3	42.4	25.4
Sub-Saharan Africa	80	199	4.1	36.8	31.5	14.0
Nigeria	71	199	2.4	14.5	75.2	8.6

Source: Adapted from Global Burden of Disease Health Financing Collaborator Network, Past, present, and future of global health financing: A review of development assistance, government, out-of-pocket, and other private spending on health for 195 countries, 1995–2050. *Lancet* 2019; 393: 2233–60. Published Online April 25, 2019. https://www.thelancet.com/journals/lancet/article/PIIS0140-6736(19)30841-4/fulltext.

shows the state of play in the run up to the most intensive discussions about issues as explored in this chapter.

The facts are stark: compared to other countries grouped by income, Nigeria spends less than most countries as a percentage of its Gross Domestic Product (GDP). This deficiency is neither recent nor a product of some dramatic economic contraction. It is a long-running pattern as indicated in Table 7.4 on the health budget in relation to the total budget at the Federal level. To the extent that health expenditure as percentage of GDP signifies commitment to invest in health outcomes and systems, Nigeria does not demonstrate seriousness of purpose when compared to its LMIC peers. To the extent that policy makers have agency, they make explicit choices in successive budget years that reflect their priorities, and those expenditures reflect their judgments of where health fits in their hierarchy of priorities.

Table 7.4. Health Sector Budget and Total Budget, 2007–2019 (NGN billions)

Year	Federal Budget	Federal Ministry of Health	Service-Wide Vote	Federal Ministry of Health + Service-Wide Vote	Federal Ministry of Health + Service-Wide Vote as % Federal Budget
FY 2007	2,266.39	123.92		123.92	5.47
FY 2008	2,992.60	144.66		144.66	4.83
FY 2009	3,557.68	154.57		154.57	4.34
FY 2010	5,159.66	169.01		169.01	3.28
FY 2011	4,484.74	257.87		257.87	5.75
FY 2012	4,877.21	284.97		284.97	5.84
FY 2013	4,987.22	282.50		282.50	5.66
FY 2014	4,695.19	264.48		264.48	5.63
FY 2015	4,493.36	259.75	2.00	261.75	5.83
FY 2016	6,060.68	250.06	3.50	253.56	4.18
FY 2017	7,441.18	308.46	3.50	311.96	4.19
FY 2018	9,120.33	356.45	58.65	415.10	4.55
FY 2019	8,826.64	365.76	75.97	441.73	5.00

Source: Akabueze B. Prioritizing health in the National Budget. Presentation at the Value for Money in the Health Sector Workshop. Director-General of the Budget Office of the Federation. March 19, 2019. Abuja.

Because the Government Health Expenditure is abysmally low and there is no viable insurance system that affords pools of pre-payment on a large scale, most of the domestic health expenditure in Nigeria is via private out-of-pocket (OOP) expenditures. This is the most regressive and least equitable form of financing, causing financial stress on households and individuals, especially the poorer segments of society. A Health Financing System Assessment[59] found that as of 2016, health insurance covered just about 4.2% of the population, and those were mostly employees of the federal government and their dependents. Consequently, OOP expenditures amounted to 75.2% of total health expenditure. This was among the highest for any country. About one quarter of households spent more than 10% of their household consumption on health.

Even the upper-middle class and the wealthy feel the consequences of a health system that does not deliver quality care: they have to seek care outside the country.[60] Nigerians of a certain vintage and those who study the country's history will recall the following:[61]

> *"One of the reasons given by the military junta when they took over power on December 31, 1983 was that the country's hospitals had become mere consulting clinics. The late Gen. Sani Abacha, who announced the coup that foisted Maj. Gen. Muhammadu Buhari on Nigerians on radio, said, 'Our economy has been hopelessly misman-aged; we have become a debtor and beggar nation... health services are in a shambles as our hospitals are reduced to mere consulting clinics without drugs, water and equipment."*

So abysmal is the situation during the second coming of Muhammadu Buhari (this time as an elected civilian President) that his own revealed preference, 35 years later, is to repeatedly seek care in the United Kingdom, where hospitals have drugs, water, and equipment.[62] That preference is a scaring indictment of the collective performance of all the governments since the messianic pretensions of the military coup in 1983.

Who is responsible for this appalling situation? Let us consider the usual suspects. It is not the "will of God," regardless of the mind-numbing penchant for organized religion that so dominates earthly discussions in Nigeria via "Shuffering and Shmiling."[63] Anyone who thinks the British deserve accolades for stiff upper lips should study the daily fortitude of the poor and marginalized people in Nigeria. The Nigerian masses seem to have perfected a phenomenon in which people put up with severe dys-functions and impunity in just about every basic public service and infra-structure here on earth while keeping faith in the possibility of a glorious hereafter. The irony is that the leaders of organized religions, who gener-ally live comfortable lives in Nigeria, evidently don't practice delayed gratification in matters like access to potable water, electricity, and quality health services. I have written elsewhere about this syndrome.[25] So, if it is not the fault of the divine, might it be that of Frederick Lugard? No, he is long gone and the British do not have to answer for this. Having eliminated the prime suspects, we are left with those supposedly cruel purveyors of global malice, the international financial institutions — the IMF and the World Bank. Can they serve as the whipping boys on this occasion?

Reasonable people might debate the legacy of the austerity measures of the mid- to late-1980s, which were promoted by the IMF and the World Bank and adopted, via a political sleight of hand, by the military junta of Ibrahim Babangida during the era of structural adjustment. As reported by Alubo:[64]

"During the last two years of the civilian government (of 1979–83), negotiation for a $2.5 billion IMF support loan was initiated. The negotiations were, however, stalled because of the anticipated political costs of the conditionality (devaluation, withdrawal of subsidies and trade liberalization) the IMF demanded. Rather than bow to these pressures, the government chose fiscal measures to conserve foreign exchange.[65]

The negotiations with the IMF continued during the 20 months of the Buhari (military) government. Again, the conditionality, particularly devaluation, was resisted. The government continued the fiscal measures of its predecessor, in addition to counter trade, i.e., the direct exchange of oil for various commodities. Counter trade was, however, frowned upon by Western creditors, including the IMF and World Bank, whose support the government needed to maintain credit facilities.[66]

The Babangida regime has now changed this situation. Irrespective of the popular rejection of the IMF loan in a national debate, the government has surreptitiously taken the loan. Since 1986, Nigeria has been implementing the IMF–World Bank prescribed austerity program. Accordingly, the currency has been devalued through public action by over 500 percent, while subsidies on petroleum, fertilizer and other products have been lifted.

The Babangida government, however, denies that it is implementing any IMF or World Bank program. It insists that the austerity programs are home grown. The ability of the government to successfully manipulate the Nigerian people has earned Babangida the sobriquet 'Maradona of Nigeria,' after the Argentinian soccer star Diego Maradona, famous for dribbling."

The truth is that through cuts in public expenditures, the combination of a collapse of oil prices in 1986 and Structural Adjustment[67] was very bad for the health and education sectors in Nigeria. Some human experiences last longer than the fleeting effects of inconclusive and highly caveated reviews by distant analysts.[68] As a young physician at the Lagos University Teaching Hospital, I witnessed many instances of patients being prematurely discharged because they could not pay the out-of-pocket user fees.

The superior truth is that the recent and current cohorts of policy makers across the executive and legislative branches of government cannot credibly hide behind the Structural Adjustment of three decades ago as the cause of their failures to accord to health — and thus to human capital development — the priorities that wise and far-sighted leaders in the Western Region of Nigeria did in the mid-1950s, and that leaders in many other countries have done elsewhere over the decades. External "partners," especially some histrionic NGOs and self-appointed fixers of Nigeria's problems from the Global North, who blame outside forces for today's policy failures in Nigeria, do the country a disservice. Their mindless advocacy, platitudinal bromides, and performative expressions of concern at the UN General Assembly (UNGA), Annual and Spring Meetings of the World Bank and the IMF, Board Meetings of the GFATM and GAVI, and various replenishment sessions for global funding entities do nothing but infantilize policy makers, gloss over Nigerians' own agency for domestic decisions, and give cover for executive ineptitude and impunity. To be utterly clear:

In the 21st century, Nigeria's leaders and policy makers have mostly chosen to neglect investments in health. No external party forced them to make those choices.

7.6. From Legislating to Budgeting

There is something striking about the display of Mercedes-Benz limousines at the entrance to the National Assembly Complex, which houses the Senate and House of Representatives in Abuja. So big and shiny are the vehicles, and so many are those taking care of the big cars, that the casual observer might wonder whether this was the flagship showroom of

Daimler-Benz in Stuttgart or a franchise of the Geneva Motor Show. But Abuja is not only physically far from Europe, it is institutionally distant and outperforms Germany and Switzerland in the yawning gap between legislative grandiosity and legislative performance. How so? It is important to examine the convergence of three important developments in health financing.

The first development was the National Health Act of 2014, which followed six decades of policy statements, legislation, and development plans.[58] The Act stipulates the following in Part I, Article 11:

(1) There is established the Basic Health Care Provision Fund (in this Act referred to as "the Fund").
(2) The Basic Health Care Provision Fund shall be financed from:
    (a) Federal Government annual grant of not less than one per cent of its Consolidated Revenue Fund;
    (b) grants by international donor partners; and
    (c) funds from any other source.

The second development was Nigeria's transition from low to lower middle-income status in 2008 and its subsequent classification as an IDA-IBRD blend country, which would limit its future eligibility for grants, cheap credits, and debt relief. Based on a GNI per capita income threshold of US$1,026 in 2015, Nigeria was one of 34 countries that made such transitions in the 20-year period that ended in 2015.[59] This transition had implications for their health financing realities. Total health spending per capita generally rises with GNI per capita. As GNI per capita grows, it is common for the portion of health finance based on pre-paid financing (like insurance) and general budgets (from tax revenues) to increase, and for OOP spending to decrease as shares of total health spending. The combination of increasing GNI per capita and decreasing eligibility for external grants and cheap credits is part of what is sometimes called *the health financing transition*. But countries often do not manage this transition well; they do not establish fair and sustainable health financing systems that can survive when the foreign aid cushion of DAH tapers off. Several colleagues and I have studied and reached some striking conclusions about the economic transition of health in Africa.[69] Nigeria, among some other countries, faces serious challenges in its health financing transition.

The passage of the National Health Act of 2014 was a landmark, but the National Assembly did not pass a budget to fulfill the stipulations of the law that was within its own purview; specifically, the provision on a Federal Government annual grant of at least 1% of its Consolidated Revenue Fund. That inaction amidst under-funding of the health sector led to considerable agitation among Nigerian health policy analysts within the country and expressions of concern by some actors in the Abuja offices of external agencies working on health in the country.

The third important development was the appointment in 2015 of Professor Isaac Adewole, formerly Vice-Chancellor of the University of Ibadan, as Minister of Health, following the election of Muhammadu Buhari as President that year. I had met Adewole many years earlier while working as Associate Director of the AIDS Prevention Initiative in Nigeria, a program funded by the Bill and Melinda Gates Foundation via a grant to the Harvard School of Public Health. Professor Phyllis Kanki, a professor of immunology and infectious disease, who combined her intellectual leadership with steely determination and a great sense of humor, led the program. Adewole, a professor of obstetrics and gynecology, combined a quiet demeanor with the political savvy to navigate the waters of the university where he was based at the time of our joint work. He wrote a chapter of the book entitled *AIDS in Nigeria*,[70] which Kanki and I coedited with Oluwole Odutolu and John Idoko. In his capacity as Minister, and in my capacity as Director of the Health, Nutrition, and Population Global Practice of the World Bank, we shared a professional interest in enabling a robust health financing system in Nigeria. It was an opportunity to break new grounds in a very challenging theater.

Many people the world over are familiar with announcements of grants, credits, and loans by the World Bank. That financing is important and often attracts the ire of some external observers and activists. What rarely makes the headlines of newspapers is the combination of analytical and advisory services — *the knowledge and know-how* — that the World Bank brings to its engagement with country officials and institutions. When country leaders recognize that they have a problem and are willing to explore informed options, customize solutions that fit their specific realities, and own the leadership challenge, the effect can be very positive. But, in my experience across the world, there are four factors required for successful collaboration:

- that country leaders truly recognize and own their own problems;
- that external analysts and advisors have the humility to study and understand the social narratives of the countries in addition to the technical dimensions of problems and potential solutions;
- that external analysts and advisors are willing and able to effectively communicate what country leaders and policy analysts need to know and consider, not pander to them by telling them what they might prefer to hear; and
- that country leaders fully own the policy decisions that they make, including the upsides and downsides.

Adewole knew his problems and I, with a superb team of specialists in health systems and economics based in Abuja and Washington DC, was going to enable frank and substantive work to inform policy options and improve the system. The government would make its own decisions. For coalition building, the Abuja-based members of the World Bank Health Team for Nigeria engaged with a wider group of country representatives of "Development Partners" from multiple agencies including multilateral organizations, bilateral agencies, and foundations.

Over the next four years, Adewole led a determined but tortuous charge to expand and rationalize the financing of health in Nigeria across the dimensions of revenue generation, pooling, allocation, and expenditures. It is a difficult task in any situation and doubly so in the complexity of Nigeria. I recall some early experiences in our work. A session with his team and key external agencies in Abuja marked the real start of the joint exercise. It was a wide-ranging discussion of financing, service delivery coverage, the capacity of the system, near-term challenges, and medium-term prospects. The second day coincided with Local Government Elections in the Abuja area, with restrictions on the movement of vehicles starting early in the morning. Adewole pledged to arrive at the meeting hall very early in the morning before the restrictions started and exhorted his team of senior FMOH officials to do the same. That was a small but important signal that the work on financing and service delivery for UHC was especially important and he expected his team to behave accordingly.

There were inevitable tensions among interest groups in terms of just what "priorities" meant. We had to distinguish between two considerations. One was the bigger picture of securing additional funds for health services *and* ensuring more effective and efficient use of those funds with probity. The other consisted of items of importance to specific constituencies — specific diseases, specific demographics, specific geographic areas, specific indicators dictated by the head offices of some bilateral agencies to their country representatives, and so on. The decision was simple: a relentless focus on the bigger picture while acknowledging, understanding, and keeping an open mind about the interests of those stakeholders. Background analyses, just-in-time technical briefs, and small-group discussions helped to build a degree of informed consensus around the challenges and options most likely to have positive multiplier effects across the system while building a platform to reduce the constraints on achieving specific objectives of interest to those stakeholders.

On October 30, 2017, Vice-President Yemi Osinbajo convened and chaired a meeting of the Federal Government's Economic Management Team, with the theme of "Investing in our people: health as a catalyzing force for economic recovery and growth" in Nigeria. It was held at the Aso Rock Complex of the Nigerian Presidency, to which I led the delegation from the World Bank. The Vice-President, who calmly led the session with curiosity and incisive questioning, enabled a very candid conversation. The immediate outcomes of the meeting were (i) a commitment by the Vice-President to take seriously the requests from the Minister of Health, (ii) a convergence on funding the basics, (iii) a convergence on pursuing an explicitly pluralistic approach to domestic revenue mobilization for health — from general revenues and contributory health insurance in ways that would make sense in Nigeria; (iv) a keen interest in developing a basic health care provision card or similar — and deploying it in a phased manner, and (v) a request from the Economic Management Team to the Minister of Health for a specific request for the

2018 budget. The Minister of Health responded to the request on the same day.

The commitment of the Executive Branch of Government was essential but not sufficient, as it is the legislative branch that passes the budget. Thus, a concurrent front for engagement consisted of the health and budget committees of the Senate and the House of Representatives. At their request, the World Bank's health team played a major role in generating and sharing with the committee leaders relevant information on health financing, inequities, inefficiencies, pilot project successes, and options for their consideration. One fortunate coincidence was that Senator Lanre Tejuosho (who was Chair of the Senate Committee on Health) and I had been colleagues as young physicians at the Lagos University Teaching Hospital, some 30 years earlier. That shared experience provided an opening to respectfully convey some hard facts about what the legislators could do about the terrible situation of health and its financing in Nigeria. To his credit, Tejuosho, in concert with others like Senator Mao Ohuabunwa, who chaired the Senate Committee on Primary Health Care and Communicable Diseases, rose to the occasion and mobilized his colleagues to find the will to pass a budget.

It is worth examining within the bigger picture a microcosm of the systemic failures, which Hafez carefully reported in the Nigeria Health System Financing Assessment.[71] Two of the many findings were especially important:

(1) In 2016, Nigeria's revenue as a share of GDP was 4.8%, and that was the poorest revenue mobilization effort of any country.

(2) "In 2016, external resources amounted to N285 billion (US$1 billion) — almost half as much as the GON spends on health — or 7.6% of total health expenditure (Federal Republic of Nigeria, 2017). Funds are predominantly from a few institutions — the International Development Association (IDA), the Global Fund to fight AIDS, tuberculosis, and malaria (GF), the United States Agency for International Development (USAID), and the Global Vaccine Alliance (Gavi). As many of these institutions have policies on transition or 'graduation,' Nigeria's health financing transition will have a significant impact on its ability to access donor aid in the future."

Where government does not step in to make up for the loss of DAH during transition from dependency on grants and concessional credits, the loss of funds would put additional pressure on health facilities. That, in turn, would necessitate the introduction of — or an increase in — user fees, with consequent increase in private OOP for essential health services. Thus did Nigeria face fundamental problems in its quest for a sustainable way to finance UHC.

Of importance to our consultation with legislators, Nigeria had entered Gavi's accelerated transition phase in 2017, with 5 years before it fully transitioned away from dependency on Gavi. It is noteworthy that in 2017, the very low levels of immunization led the Federal Government to declare a national emergency. The declaration of emergency about an eminently predictable need was, I thought, a feat of policy contortions. Evidently, the Government had shown little or no seriousness about graduating from dependency on the kindness of strangers, even for the most elementary responsibility: the financing of all-too-predictable routine immunization for its children.

The systemic failure went beyond immunization. One of my business trips to Nigeria coincided with a visit by officials of the African Leaders Malaria Alliance (ALMA). They were scurrying from one donor agency office in Abuja to another, seeking funds for the emergency purchase of commodities for malaria control. *How, in a malaria-endemic country that literally sits on oil, does the largely predictable need for insecticide-treated bednets become an emergency?* It is what happens when governments abdicate basic responsibilities. It is what happens when advocates for foreign aid of infinite quantities and infinite duration obfuscate instead of telling the truth. It is what happens when the citizenry put up with impunity and culpable dereliction of duty in high places. That is the construct that makes many countries of the Global South the laughing stock of the Global North. A long-time colleague in the profession put it this way in pidgin English: *"Dem no dey shame."*[b]

In March 2018, a multiagency delegation visited Nigeria to consult with government officials on the challenge of financing vaccines for

---

[b] They have no shame.

routine immunization. Dr. Seth Berkley, CEO of Gavi (The Vaccine Alliance, whose *raison d'etre* is to enable the sustainable financing of vaccines), led the delegation in which I participated on behalf of the World Bank. The global landscape is rife with examples of failure to graduate from dependency on foreign aid for essential services. I resolved to do all I could to ensure that this particular engagement did not become yet another hollow ritual in which donors pretended to be serious and country officials pretended to take them seriously.

Now, back to those Mercedes-Benz limousines at the National Assembly Complex in Abuja, which were purchased with the "people's money," the people being the millions of Nigerians whose access to routine vaccines depended on the fickle kindness of strangers from thousands of miles away. There was something jarring, even grotesque, about the juxtaposition of those limousines with a consultation about the country's failure to finance routine vaccines for its own children. It was pathetic in a very fundamental way. Having passed the security screening process, our delegation made its way past a hallway with photographs of those who led the country to independence and ruled it in the first republic.

The meeting with a group of Senators and members of the House of Representatives began with warm greetings. Several of the people, if not old colleagues or friends, were familiar from earlier consultations on the broader topic of UHC and health financing in the country. With the opening pitch by Berkley and some initial discussions over, I decided that it was time to cut to the essence of the problem.

"Thank you for taking the time to meet with us, honorable Senators and members of the House of Representatives. It is an honor to be here. Walking into this meeting today, we passed a hall with photographs of historical leaders of this country around the time of independence. But what does independence mean? It means taking responsibility for one's affairs. I doubt that when Nigeria achieved independence, its leaders meant for it to permanently depend on the kindness of strangers for the basic necessities of its children. Vaccines are basic necessities. Yet, here we are. Imagine a man who does not feed his children, who does not buy books for his children in primary school, who goes around

begging others to feed his family. Imagine that same man buying Mercedes-Benz cars, displaying them outside his house, and inviting his neighbors to admire those cars. That is where Nigeria is as a country.

About 50 years ago, Martin Luther King, Jr., challenged his country to 'Be true to what you said on paper.' You, honorable Senators and members of the House of Representatives, passed the National Health Act of 2014. But you have not passed a budget to back it up. I respectfully ask you to be true to what you said on paper. If you cannot do it just to stop Nigeria from continuing as a beggar on the world stage, you can do it as a service to the children of this country. But do it you must. A self-respecting and sovereign nation should not permanently depend on the kindness of strangers for the most basic things. Thank you."

There was a brief silence in the room, followed by promises by the legislators to make things happen. We parted with smiles, handshakes, some hugs, and a shared knowledge that the era of evasive platitudes and euphemisms was over.

My delivery was not a spontaneous act. I had honed it and recently delivered essentially the same messages in a public forum, as the Keynote Speech at the first *ThisDay* Health Financing Forum on March 6, 2018. My phone starting ringing almost nonstop, with calls from senior officials and former colleagues. Most were thankful that someone finally cut through the static to say what needed to be said in the public domain. A tiny minority urged me to leave things alone because Nigerians did not want to hear the truth. I thanked the former group and told the latter group that, with all due respect, nothing would change unless each of us summoned the courage, in our different places, to change things.

Vice-President Yemi Osinbajo met with our delegation. I regarded this as a mark of his own seriousness of purpose. Whereas our first meeting in 2017 was on system-wide issues and options for financing the health system, the focus on this occasion was on the narrower — but important — topic of vaccines and how Nigeria would graduate from Gavi financing.

The legislators delivered on their promise. In May 2018, the National Assembly finally passed a budget that included provisions envisaged in the National Health Act of 2014. Sometimes, quiet satisfaction is the best celebration. It felt good. Deep inside, I dedicated that little success to the millions who had suffered from poor or unaffordable health care in Nigeria, and especially to those patients who had been prematurely discharged from hospital because their families could not afford the fees. I was in the office when the message came from Abuja. It was a sunny day in Washington DC. I stepped outside, crossed the street and took a ten-minute walk around Lafayette Square in front of the White House. There were the usual tourists, a few people with placards promoting their causes, secret service agents, and people just going about their lives. Each of them probably had strong views about the vagaries of health financing in the United States, but they probably had no idea about what it was like to be at the mercy of unaffordable health costs in Nigeria. To paraphrase Leo Tolstoy, every happy health system is happy in the same way, but each unhappy health system is unhappy in its own way.

The consultations also resulted in an agreement to finance vaccines and Gavi Counterpart funds via a Service-Wide Vote item in the budget, in addition to the budget channeled through the Federal Ministry of Health. According to the Budget Office of the Federation, the aggregate budget for immunization increased by 158% from NGN12 billion in 2018 to NGN31 billion in 2019 via additional funding for vaccines through the Service-Wide Vote.[72]

7.7. From Budgeting to Implementation

Passing a budget is a legislative statement of intent and commitment to relative priorities. Spending the money on time, effectively, and efficiently is a monumental challenge in Nigeria. The National Health Act of 2014, which stipulated the creation of a Basic Health Care Provision Fund (BHCPF), stated what the Fund would finance on the demand and the supply sides of health services (quoted in Box 7.1).[73]

Box 7.1. What the Basic Health Care Provision Fund Would Finance

(3) Money from the Fund shall be used to finance the following:

    (a) 50 percent of the Fund shall be used for the provision of basic minimum package of health services to citizens, in eligible primary or secondary health care facilities through the National Health Insurance Scheme (NHIS);

    (b) 20 percent of the Fund shall be used to provide essential drugs, vaccines, and consumables for eligible primary health care facilities;

    (c) 15 percent of the Fund shall be used for the provision and maintenance of facilities, equipment, and transport for eligible primary health care facilities; and

    (d) 10 percent of the Fund shall be used for the development of human resources for primary health care; and

    (e) 5 percent of the Fund shall be used for emergency medical treatment to be administered by a Committee appointed by the National Council on Health.

(4) The National Primary Health Care Development Agency shall disburse the funds for subsection 3 (b), (c) and (d) of this section through State and Federal Capital Territory Primary Health Care Boards for distribution to Local Government and Area Council Health Authorities.

(5) For any State or Local Government to qualify for a block grant pursuant to sub-section (1) of this section, such State or Local Government shall contribute:

    (a) in the case of a State, not less than 25 percent of the total of projects; and

    (b) in the case of a Local Government, not less than 25 percent of the total cost of projects as their commitment in the execution of such projects.

(6) The National Primary Health Care Development Agency shall not disburse money to any:

    (a) Local Government Health Authority if it is not satisfied that the money earlier disbursed was applied in accordance with the provisions of the Act;

    (b) State or Local Government that fails to contribute its counterpart funding; and

    (c) States and Local Governments that fail to implement the national health policy, norms, standards and guidelines prescribed by the National Council on Health.

Thus, the BHCPF is a statutory federal program, intended to provide an additional source of financing that was primarily aimed at front line health service providers.[74] To be effective, it required not only an initial capitalization but also decision-enabling data on health spending and resource flows, including the cost and use of health services. The Operation Manual of the BHCPF, which provided detailed guidelines for its implementation via three gateways, was first issued in 2018,[75] and revised in 2020.[76] The 2020 version provides in detail the governance structure and operations of each of the Gateways, and fiduciary measures and sanctions. More specifically:

- The sections relating to the NPHCDA Gateway outline roles and responsibilities for the NPHCDA, the State PHC Boards and Agencies, the Local Government Health Authorities (LGHAs), Ward Development Committees (WDCs), and PHC facilities.
- The sections on the NHIS Gateway outline how Nigerians and health care providers would enroll to become beneficiaries of the BHCPF, which would enable citizens to access care based on the Basic Minimum Package of Health Services (BMPHS) at no cost to them in designated PHC and secondary health facilities. The key opportunity here is the pursuit of strategic purchasing reforms, which would both improve accountability and provide an opportunity to better engage the private sector in service delivery.
- Bridging the gap between need and access to health care in emergency situations is the Emergency Medical Treatment (EMT) Gateway managed by the National EMT Committee as appointed by the National Council on Health.

There are four prominent challenges, among many others, in the approach to financing via the BHCPF and to the approach to implementation noted above.

- First, although the BHCPF is a predominantly tax-financed construct, expectations of increasing allocations to health, even if 1% were allocated every year, are only as good as the increases in the denominator, the Federal Consolidated Revenue Fund. According to the World Bank, the macroeconomic situation has deteriorated beyond the situation in 2015–2016, when oil prices fell and the Nigerian economy went into recession for the first time in 25 years. Nigeria now has fewer buffers and policy instruments to cushion adverse effects.[77]

Since additional general revenues will be hard to come by in the immediate future, it is especially important to squeeze as much value as possible from the revenues coming to health, both as a matter of good practice and in the pursuit of progressive realization of UHC. The BHCPF has the additional merit of being a *de facto* public financial management reform as it provides an accountability framework to ensure that resources get to the frontline of service delivery. This potential is tempered by the fact that the combination of health financing and public financial management reforms requires additional technical capacity for its implementation at the federal and state levels.

- Second, it is suboptimal to continue an approach of paying for PHC services that is mostly based on inputs and processes, instead of being based on some locally customized combination of outcomes, outputs, and quality-assured processes. The former risks perpetuating inefficiencies, with no incentives to nudge service providers toward higher performance. It also risks a failure to scale up and improve upon the very positive lessons learned from performance-based financing in Nigeria, especially under the Nigeria State Health Investment Project (NSHIP). The NSHIP, at its core, is a decentralized financing facility, which enables primary health care facilities to use funds received for much needed improvements for service delivery. There is no point in expecting high-quality services without giving the frontline staff in charge of those facilities the resources needed for better performance. The following is noteworthy as a home-grown alternative to the antiquated and input-driven approach:[59]

"The NSHIP facilities significantly improved key aspects of PHC performance. A randomized impact evaluation found that after more than 30 months of implementation, participating NSHIP facilities increased coverage of pentavalent vaccine by 15 percentage points, facility births by 9 percentage points, and modern contraceptive prevalence by 7 percentage points compared with the status quo — all at the relatively

modest cost of $1.20 per capita per year. Furthermore, NSHIP improved quality of care in 49 percent of facilities."

- Third, there remains a continuing lack of clarity about just what the NHIS can accomplish with specific reference to the aspects of its revenue that derive from premiums (i.e., revenue from sources other than the BHCPF). Health insurance is not viable in the absence of a willingness and capacity to enforce contributions, and without a capacity to collect premiums from subscribers in the informal sector. In a context with high rates of poverty and informality in the economy, it is not realistic to regard insurance, *especially labor-tax financed social health insurance*, as a viable way for governments to avoid paying from general revenues for health services needed by large parts of the population. Yet, the situation in Nigeria is tenuous with regard to tax base, etc. The conceptual and practical challenges with which Nigeria must contend are well documented in the literature.[78–80] The government needs to: enforce the payroll contribution of 1.75% of the consolidated salary of federal civil servants (the employees' contribution); rationalize the number and size of risk pools; define the scale and type of risk-moderating mechanisms that will reduce inequalities in health financing across states; rationalize the size and types of administrative costs; determine which government (e.g., Federal or State) will subsidize the payment of insurance premiums for the poor in mandatory schemes; and professionalize the management of the NHIS.

The NHIS was established in 1999 by the decree of a military government. Its challenges arise from a combination of congenital defects, design problems, and execution problems. A military decree had the explicit and implicit expectation of a command-and-control approach to implementation — one in which all the states and citizens would comply with the NHIS act. When implementation started in 2005, only very few states signed up to the health insurance program as envisaged under the NHIS Act of 1999. The NHIS was unable to expand coverage beyond employees of the federal government. Meaningful reforms had to include some degree of decentralization of health insurance functions to states. Whilst this was a second best option with its attendant transaction costs, there was no obvious path for progress in a single risk pool because several states were not convinced that they had to be part of a single national health insurance pool.

In 2015, the NHIS, with the support of the World Bank/IFC advisory program, adopted a memorandum that granted Nigerian states the ability to set up their State Supported Health Insurance Agencies (SSHIAs).[81] Furthermore, the implementation of the BHCPF of the National Health Act of 2014 (i.e., NHIS Gateway) would have been impractical without having the state-owned health insurance schemes in place. The start of the BHCPF in 2019 further nudged state governments to establish their SSHIAs. As of the first quarter of 2021, most Nigerian states had set up their state insurance agencies, with the exception of Rivers State. However, the formal establishment of SSHIAs is only a step in a series of essential actions, including but not limited to: identification and enrolment of the poor and vulnerable; defining and costing of the benefit package; release of funds by the state government to cover the poor and vulnerable; accreditation and enrollment of both public and private providers; and reimbursement of providers upon the delivery of services. In addition, it is crucial to ensure that health facilities can deliver services to the insured, otherwise the insurance schemes would lose credibility.

- Fourth is the challenge of how to make the best use of the widespread private sector service delivery facilities and supply chains. This is a longstanding and unresolved problem. In 2007, a review of the private sector and existing Public–Private Partnerships (PPPs) found huge but unexplored opportunities for harnessing the private sector to improve PHC services through PPPs.[82] The authors suggested three broad strategies: making productive use of existing private sector providers; encouraging private providers to expand services to underserved populations or areas; and taking advantage of the comparative strength of the private sector. The current landscape of PPPs is fragmented, and that fragmentation is further complicated by the dearth of truly strategic purchasing by the public sector. There are several models in operation:[83]

o Large-scale hospital PPP/Integrated model, such as the Cancer Center PPP between the Lagos University Teaching Hospital and the Nigeria Sovereign Investment Authority (NSIA).

o Hospital Management Contracts, with private entities managing the Garki General Hospital in Abuja and the Ibom Specialist Hospital in Akwa Ibom State.

o Limited Hospital PPP/Discrete Clinical Services Model: Several Federal Government-owned teaching hospitals have contracted out their radiology units and one of them has contracted out its pathology laboratory since 2009.

o PPPs for PHC: Several state governments have contracted existing PHC centers to private operators.

o PPPs for Public Health Services: An example is the agreement between MDS Logistics and the Federal Government/FMOH for the "Warehouse in a box."

Progress on the PPP front will require an astute combination of global principles and local realities.[84]

7.8. Looking Ahead

Despite the array of problems, Nigeria still has opportunities for the progressive realization of UHC. But success is not guaranteed. Progress will depend on two crucial dimensions: changes within the country and changes in the architecture and practice of foreign aid.

Possibly the most important change within the country is the elevation of an effective health system to a matter of serious importance with consequences for elected officials. If a government cannot provide credible evidence that it is making a serious effort to make essential health services available and affordable, the people should vote the government out of office. Individual legislators at the Federal, State, and Local Government levels need to face similar scrutiny of their work, with the consequence for poor performance being losing their next elections.

Much will depend on how well governments at the federal and state levels learn and act upon lessons from the COVID-19 pandemic. At the federal level, early indications are suggestive of more wisdom in financing health. For example, there is a realization that a massive health emergency can rapidly become a fiscal emergency and that investing in preparedness could be less costly than responding. This led to a proposed increase in the capital allocation to the Federal Ministry of Health by 82% from the revised 2020 budget of NGN51.4 billion to NGN93.68 billion in 2021.[85] However, these are still early days, and it remains to be seen whether the searing experience of COVID-19, which laid bare the shoddy state of the health system, will result in lasting commitments to change.

Another consideration is to use a combination of equity-enhancing mechanisms for raising revenues. This is primarily from general revenues, secondarily from health insurance that includes public subsidies for the poor, and from pro-health taxes on tobacco, alcohol, and sugar-sweetened beverages.[86,87]

More specific needs for change within the country, which I have addressed elsewhere in the literature, include the following:[25]

(a) Public accountability for basic health services and public goods, with a backbone of public financial management and transparency;
(b) A credible, professional, and effective health planning, finance, and metrics function in the federal and state ministries of health;
(c) A shift to performance-based financing of essential health services (to which should be added direct facility financing, in light of new evidence on this mechanism[88]);
(d) Better use of the private sector for supply chains and clinical service delivery;
(e) Development of institutions for core public health functions; and
(f) Channeling civil society activism and the emerging accountability paradigm.

The second dimension is the nature and focus of DAH. Two decades into the 21st century, there is a need for major shifts in thinking and practice. Most of the necessary changes are not unique to Nigeria and will be examined in more detail in Chapter 8, on the real-world dynamics of DAH.

References

[1] Crowder M. 1962. *The Story of Nigeria*. London: Faber and Faber. 416 pp.

[2] Perham M. Frederick Lugard. British colonial administrator. https://www.britannica.com/biography/Frederick-Lugard. Accessed on February 14, 2021.

[3] Rodney W. 2011. *How Europe Underdeveloped Africa*. Black Classic Press. Paperback: 340 pages.

[4] Pakenham T. 1991. *The Scramble for Africa. The White Man's Conquest of the Dark Continent from 1876 to 1912*. New York: Random House.

[5] Bolton G. 2007. *Africa Doesn't Matter. How the West Has Failed the Poorest Continent and What We Can Do About It*. New York: Arcade Publishing. 350 pp.

[6] Shillington K. 1989. *History of Africa*. New York: St. Martin's Press.

[7] Khan WN. The Atlantic slave trade and its lasting impact. In Levan AC, Ukata (Editors). *The Oxford Handbook of Nigerian Politics*. Oxford University Press. pp. 60–74.

[8] Hochschild A. 1998. *King Leopold's Ghost: A Story of Greed, Terror, and Heroism in Colonial Africa*. First Mariner Books. 366 pp.

[9] Igbafe PA. 1970. The fall of Benin: A reassessment. *The Journal of African History*, 11(3): 385–400. https://www.jstor.org/stable/180345?seq=1. Accessed on February 14, 2021.

[10] Akinjogbin IA. 1966. The Oyo Empire in the 18th century — A reassessment. *Journal of the Historical Society of Nigeria*. 3(3): 449–460. https://www.jstor.org/stable/41856706. Accessed on February 14, 2021.

[11] Health Reform Foundation of Nigeria. 2007. *Nigeria Health Review*. Abuja, Nigeria: HERFON. pp. 1–10.

[12] WHO called to return to the Declaration of Alma-Ata International conference on primary health care. https://www.who.int/teams/social-determinants-of-health/declaration-of-alma-ata#:~:text=Primary%20health%20care%20is%20essential,afford%20to%20maintain%20at%20every. Accessed on February 15, 2021.

[13] United Nations General Assembly. Political declaration of the high-level meeting on universal health coverage. Resolution adopted by the General Assembly on October 10, 2019. p. 1. https://undocs.org/en/A/RES/74/2. Accessed on February 15, 2021.

[14] Aregbeshola BS, Khan SM. 2017. Primary health care in Nigeria: 24 years after Olikoye Ransome-Kuti's leadership. *Frontiers in Public Health*, 13 March. https://doi.org/10.3389/fpubh.2017.00048. Accessed on February 15, 2021.

[15] Fatusi AO. Public health leadership, policy development and the Nigerian health system. *A Paper Presented at the Induction Program of the Institute for Government Research Leadership Technology.* Abuja: (2015). Available from: http://www.instituteforgovernmentresearch.org/images/abuja2015g/abuja2015. docx.

[16] Ransome-Kuti O. 1998. *Who Cares for the Health of Africans?: The Nigerian Case' International Lecture Series on Population Issues.* Kaduna, Nigeria: The John D. and Catherine T. MacArthur Foundation. Available from: http://www. popline.org/node/525102.

[17] Lambo E. 2015. Primary health care: Realities, challenges and the way forward. *A Paper Presented at the First Annual Primary Health Care Lecture.* Abuja. Available from: http://nigeriahealthwatch.com/wp-content/uploads/bsk-pdf-manager/1160_2015_Primary_Health_Care_Presentation_Final,_NPHCDA_1216. pdf.

[18] Lucas AO. 2010. *It Was the Best of Times: From Local to Global Health.* Ibadan, Nigeria: Book Builders. pp. 333–335.

[19] Health Reform Foundation of Nigeria. 2008. Nigerian health review 2007. *Primary Health Care in Nigeria: 30 Years after Alma Ata.* Abuja. Nigeria.

[20] Gyuse AN, Ayuk AE, Okeke MC. 2018. Facilitators and barriers to effective primary health care in Nigeria. *African Journal of Primary Health Care & Family Medicine*, 10(1): a1641. https://www.ncbi.nlm.nih.gov/pmc/articles/PMC5843931/. Accessed on February 15, 2021.

[21] Oyekale AS. 2017. Assessment of primary health care facilities' service readiness in Nigeria. BMC Health Services Research, 17, Article number: 172. https:// bmchealthservres.biomedcentral.com/articles/10.1186/s12913-017-2112-8. Accessed on February 15, 2021.

[22] World Bank. 2008. *Nigeria—Improving Primary Health Care Delivery: Evidence from Four States.* Washington, DC. World Bank. https://openknowledge. worldbank.org/handle/10986/7784. Accessed on February 15, 2021.

[23] Kress DH, Su Y, Wang H. 2016. Assessment of primary health care system performance in Nigeria: Using the primary health care performance indicator conceptual framework. *Health Systems and Reform.* https://www.tandfonline.com/doi/full/10.1080/23288604.2016.1234861. Accessed on June 8, 2021.

[24] World Bank. *Nigeria — Immunization Plus and Malaria Progress by Accelerating Coverage and Transforming Services Project* (English). Washington, D.C.: World Bank Group. http://documents.worldbank.org/curated/ en/102621580321213128/Nigeria-Immunization-Plus-and-Malaria-Progress-by-Accelerating-Coverage-and-Transforming-Services-Project. Accessed on February 17, 2021.

[25] Adeyi O. 2016. Health in Nigeria: From underperformance to measured optimism. *Health Systems and Reform*, 2(4): 285–289. https://www.tandfonline.com/doi/full/10.1080/23288604.2016.1224023. Accessed on February 17, 2021.

[26] Babalola S., Fatusi A. 2009. Determinants of use of maternal health services in Nigeria — looking beyond individual and household factors. *BMC Pregnancy and Childbirth*, 9: 43. http://bmcpregnancychildbirth.biomedcentral.com/articles/10.1186/1471-2393-9-43. Accessed on February 17, 2021.

[27] Onwuameze NC. 2013. Educational opportunity and inequality in Nigeria: Assessing social background, gender and regional effects. Doctoral dissertation. http://ir.uiowa.edu/cgi/viewcontent.cgi?article=4727&context=etd. Accessed on February 17, 2021.

[28] Adetoro JE. 1966. Universal primary education and the teacher supply problem in Nigeria. *Comparative Education*, 2(3): 209–216. https://www.tandfonline.com/doi/abs/10.1080/0305006660020307. Accessed on February 17, 2021.

[29] World Bank. The human capital index 2020 update: Human capital in the time of COVID-19. https://openknowledge.worldbank.org/handle/10986/34432. Accessed on February 18, 2021.

[30] World Bank. 2003. *World Development Report 2004: Making Services Work for Poor People*. Washington, DC: World Bank and Oxford University Press. pp. 46–63.

[31] Okonjo-Iweala N. 2012. *Reforming the Unreformable: Lessons from Nigeria*. Cambridge: The MIT Press. pp. 81–94.

[32] Isiguzo I. Covid-19 exposes how Prof Odekunle's powerful friends see Nigeria. 2021. https://businessday.ng/opinion/article/covid-19-exposes-how-prof-odekunles-powerful-friends-see-nigeria/ Accessed on February 18, 2021.

[33] Mmonu NA, Aifah A, Onakomaiya D, Ogedegbe G. 2021. Why the global health community should support the EndSARS movement in Nigeria. *The Lancet*. https://www.thelancet.com/action/showPdf?pii=S0140-6736%2821%2900194-X. Accessed on February 21, 2021.

[34] Smith DJ. Progress and setbacks in Nigeria's anticorruption efforts. 2018. In Levan AC, Ukata (Editors). *The Oxford Handbook of Nigerian Politics*. Oxford University Press. pp. 288–301.

[35] Achebe C. 1983. The trouble with Nigeria. Fourth Dimension Pub. Enugu. Nigeria.

[36] Smith DJ. 2007. *A Culture of Corruption: Everyday Deception and Political Discontent in Nigeria*. Princeton, NJ: Princeton University Press.

[37] Lawson L. 2009. The politics of anticorruption reform in Nigeria. *Journal of Modern African Studies*, 47(1), 79–103.

[38] Adebanwi W, Obadare E. 2011. When corruption fights back: Democracy and elite interests in Nigeria's anti-corruption war. *Journal of Modern African Studies.* 49(2): 185–213.

[39] Chabal P, Daloz JP. 1999. *Africa Works: The Political Instrumentalization of Disorder.* Bloomington, IN: Indiana University Press.

[40] Liebovich M. 2013. *This Town: Two Parties and a Funeral-Plus, Plenty of Valet Parking!-in America's Gilded Capital.* New York: Penguin Group.

[41] Whyte D. 2015. *How Corrupt Is Britain?* London: Pluto Press.

[42] Behr R. Britain believes it's free of corruption. But there's still the stench of decay. *The Guardian.* https://www.theguardian.com/commentisfree/2021/apr/13/britain-free-corruption-decay-david-cameron. Accessed on April 17, 2021.

[43] Asthana A, Grierson J. 2016. Afghanistan and Nigeria 'possibly most corrupt countries', Cameron lets slip. https://www.theguardian.com/uk-news/2016/may/10/david-cameron-afghanistan-nigeria-possibly-most-corrupt-countries. Accessed February 18, 2021.

[44] Elgot J. 2021. David Cameron breaks 30-day silence over lobbying for Greensill. https://www.theguardian.com/politics/2021/apr/11/david-cameron-breaks-silence-on-greensill-lobbying-scandal? Accessed on April 12, 2021.

[45] Kirka D. 2021. UK lobbying scandal snares ex-PM Cameron; govt starts probe. https://apnews.com/article/2f84245d4901474b07fa76c8c1053b3b. Accessed on April 12, 2021.

[46] Short S. 2016. This is the essay on corruption that David Cameron didn't want you to read. *The Independent.* https://www.independent.co.uk/voices/essay-corruption-david-cameron-didn-t-want-you-read-a7026496.html. Accessed on April 17, 2021.

[47] The Guardian Editorial. 2016. The Guardian view on corruption: David Cameron should look closer to home. https://www.theguardian.com/commentisfree/2016/may/10/the-guardian-view-on-corruption-david-cameron-should-look-closer-to-home. Accessed on April 18, 2021.

[48] Bai J, Jayachandran S, Malesky E, Olken B. Growing out of corruption. https://epod.cid.harvard.edu/article/growing-out-corruption. Accessed February 18, 2021.

[49] GFATM. 2016. Investigation in Nigeria. https://www.theglobalfund.org/en/oig/updates/2016-05-03-investigation-in-nigeria/. Accessed on February 18, 2021.

[50] GFATM. 2020. Salary fraud and abuse affecting global fund grants. https://www.theglobalfund.org/en/oig/updates/2020-02-28-salary-fraud-and-abuse-affecting-global-fund-grants/ Accessed on February 18, 2021.

[51] Onwujekwe O *et al.* 2019. Corruption in Anglophone West Africa health systems: A systematic review of its different variants and the factors that sustain

them. *Health Policy Plan*, 34(7): 529–543. https://academic.oup.com/heapol/article/34/7/529/5543565. Accessed on February 18, 2021.

[52] Tormusa D, Mogum A. 2016. The impediments of corruption on the efficiency of healthcare service delivery in Nigeria. *The Online Journal of Health Ethics*, 12(1). DOI: 10.18785/ojhe.1201.03. Accessed on February 18, 2021.

[53] World Bank. 2015. Program appraisal document on a proposed credit in the amount of SDR354.7 million (US$500 million equivalent) to the Federal Republic of Nigeria for a program-for-results to support the saving one million lives initiative. Report No. 94852-NG. World Bank. Accessed on July 24, 2016. http://www-wds.worldbank.org/external/default/WDSContentServer/WDSP/IB/2015/04/27/090224b082df8f8f/1_0/Rendered/PDF/Nigeria000Savi0ults00Pfor R00Project.pdf.

[54] Enabulele, O. My Assessment of Nigeria's health sector performance at 53. http://saharareporters.com/2013/09/30/my-assessment-nigerias-health-sector-performance-53-dr-osahon-enabulele. Accessed on August 9, 2016.

[55] Constitution of the Federal Republic of Nigeria. 1999. http://www.nigeria-law.org/ConstitutionOfTheFederalRepublicOfNigeria.htm. Accessed on August 9, 2016.

[56] Arowosegbe, JO. 2014. Techniques for division of legislative powers under federal constitutions. *Journal of Law, Policy and Globalization*, 29.

[57] Elemo OM. 2018. Fiscal federalism, subnational politics, and state creation in contemporary Nigeria. In Levan AC, Ukata (Editors). *The Oxford Handbook of Nigerian Politics*. Oxford University Press. pp. 189–204.

[58] Federal Republic of Nigeria. National Health Act 2014. Government Notice No. 208. Federal Republic of Nigeria. Official Gazette No. 145. Vol. 101. A139-172. http://www.nphcda.gov.ng/Reports%20and%20Publications/Official%20Gazette%20of%20the%20National%20Health%20Act.pdf. Accessed on July 24, 2016.

[59] Hafez R. 2018. Nigeria health system financing assessment. World Bank https://openknowledge.worldbank.org/handle/10986/30174. Accessed on February 20, 2021.

[60] VOA. 2019. Nigeria losing $1b annually to medical tourism, authorities say. https://www.voanews.com/africa/nigeria-losing-1b-annually-medical-tourism-authorities-say. Accessed on February 19, 2021.

[61] Ojoye T. 2018. Inside some Nigeria's appalling public health centres. https://punchng.com/inside-some-nigerias-appalling-public-health-centres/. Accessed on April 14, 2021.

[62] Akinwotu E. Nigeria's president draws criticism for seeking medical care abroad. 2018. https://www.nytimes.com/2018/05/08/world/africa/nigeria-president-buhari-health.html. Accessed on April 14, 2021.

[63] Anikulapo-Kuti F. Shuffering and shmiling. https://songmeanings.com/songs/view/3530822107858727846/. Accessed on February 19, 2021.

[64] Alubo SO. 1992. Health services and military messianism in Nigeria (1983–1990). *Journal of Social Development in Africa*, 7(1), 45–65. https://www.semanticscholar.org/paper/Health-Services-and-Military-Messianism-in-Nigeria-Alubo/17f7a4f27966d1a9270a129d14e8f312a3334187. Accessed on February 19, 2021.

[65] Forrest T. 1986. The political economy of civil rule and the economic crisis in Nigeria (1978–84). *Review of African Political Economy*, 35, 4–26. In Alubo SO. Health Services and Military Messianism in Nigeria (1983–1990). *Journal of Social Development in Africa*, 7(1), 45–65. https://www.semanticscholar.org/paper/Health-Services-and-Military-Messianism-in-Nigeria-Alubo/17f7a4f2796 6d1a9270a129d14e8f312a3334187. Accessed on February 19, 2021.

[66] Bangura Y. 1992. Structural adjustment and the political question. *Review of African Political Economy*. 37, 24–37. In Alubo SO. Health Services and Military Messianism in Nigeria (1983–1990). *Journal of Social Development in Africa*, 7(1): 45–65. https://www.semanticscholar.org/paper/Health-Services-and-Military-Messianism-in-Nigeria-Alubo/17f7a4f27966d1a9270a129d14e8f3 12a3334187. Accessed on February 19, 2021.

[67] World Bank. 1994. *Nigeria Structural Adjustment Program. Policies, Implementation, and Impact*. Report Number 13053-UNI. http://documents1.worldbank.org/curated/en/959091468775569769/pdf/multi0page.pdf. Accessed on February 19, 2021.

[68] van der Gaag J, Barham T. 1998. Health and health expenditures in adjusting and non-adjusting countries. *Social Science & Medicine*, 46(8): 995–1009. https://pubmed.ncbi.nlm.nih.gov/9579751/. Accessed on February 19, 2021.

[69] Ly C, Eozenou P, Nandakumar A, Pablos-Mendez A, Evans T, Adeyi O. The economic transition of health in Africa: A call for progressive pragmatism to shape the future of health financing. *Health Systems and Reform*. Published online on May 16, 2017. https://www.tandfonline.com/doi/full/10.1080/2328860 4.2017.1325549. Accessed on February 20, 2021.

[70] Adeyi O, Kanki P, Odutolu O, Idoko, J. (Editors). 2006. *AIDS in Nigeria*. Boston, MA: Harvard University Center for Population and Development Studies.

[71] Hafez R. 2018. Nigeria health system financing assessment. World Bank. https://openknowledge.worldbank.org/handle/10986/30174. Accessed on February 20, 2021.

[72] Akabueze B. 2019. Prioritizing health in the National Budget. Presentation at the Value for Money in the Health Sector Workshop. Director-General of the Budget Office of the Federation, March 19, 2019, Abuja.

[73] Federal Republic of Nigeria. National Health Act 2014. Government Notice No. 208. Federal Republic of Nigeria Official Gazette 2014; 101: A139–A172. Available at https://nigeriahealthwatch.com/wp-content/uploads/bsk-pdf-manager/2018/07/01_-Official-Gazette-of-the-National-Health-Act-FGN.pdf. Accessed on February 20, 2021.

[74] Hafez R. 2018. Nigeria health system financing assessment. World Bank. https://openknowledge.worldbank.org/handle/10986/30174. Accessed on February 20, 2021.

[75] Federal Ministry of Health (FMOH), National Health Insurance Scheme (NHIS) and the National Primary Health Care Development Agency (NPHCDA). Basic Health Care Provision Fund. Operations Manual. November 2018. Abuja, Nigeria. http://dc.sourceafrica.net/documents/120710-OPERATIONS-MAN-UAL-of-BHCPF.html Accessed on February 21, 2021.

[76] Federal Ministry of Health (FMOH), National Health Insurance Scheme (NHIS) and the National Primary Health Care Development Agency (NPHCDA). June 2020. Guideline for the Administration, Disbursement, and Monitoring of the Basic Healthcare Provision Fund. Developed by National Primary Care Development Agency (NPHCDA) in collaboration with the National Health Insurance Scheme (NHIS) and National Emergency Medical Treatment Committee (NEMTC).

[77] World Bank. Nigeria. Overview. https://www.worldbank.org/en/country/nigeria/overview. Accessed on February 20, 2021.

[78] Cotlear D *et al.* 2015. *Going Universal: How 24 countries Are Improving Universal Health Coverage Reforms from the Bottom Up*. Washington DC: The World Bank.

[79] Yazbeck A *et al.* 2020. The case against labor-tax-financed social health insurance for low- and low-middle-income countries. *Health Affairs*, 39(5). https://www.healthaffairs.org/doi/full/10.1377/hlthaff.2019.00874. Accessed on February 21, 2021.

[80] Alawode G, Adewole A. 2021. Assessment of the design and implementation challenges of the National Health Insurance Scheme in Nigeria: A qualitative study among sub-national level actors, healthcare and insurance providers. BMC

Public Health, 21, Article number: 124. https://bmcpublichealth.biomedcentral.com/articles/10.1186/s12889-020-10133-5. Accessed on February 18, 2021.

[81] Memorandum of the Honorable Minister of Health on the Implementation of State Supported Health Insurance Schemes (SSHIS). March 2015, 58th NCH Memo No.

[82] Health Reform Foundation of Nigeria. *Nigeria Health Review 2007. Private Sector and Primary Health Care in Nigeria.* Abuja, Nigeria: HERFON. pp. 255–269.

[83] Okunola O. Personal communication. February 2021.

[84] Anyaehie USB, Nwakoby B, Chikwendu C, Dim C, Uguru N, Oluka C, Ogugua C. 2014. Constraints, challenges and prospects of public-private partnership in health-care delivery in a developing economy. *Annals of Medical and Health Science Research*, 4(1): 61–66. https://pubmed.ncbi.nlm.nih.gov/24669333/. Accessed on February 22, 2021.

[85] Akabueze B. Budgeting process in Nigeria and financing health emergencies. Undated. Presentation delivered at Multi-Sectoral Workshop for Financing Health Emergencies in Nigeria. Budget Office of the Federation, Abuja.

[86] Popkin B, Ng S. 2021. Sugar-sweetened beverage taxes: Lessons to date and the future of taxation. *PLoS Medicine.* https://journals.plos.org/plosmedicine/article?id=10.1371/journal.pmed.1003412. Accessed on April 14, 2021.

[87] The Task Force on Fiscal Policy for Health. 2019. Health taxes to save lives: Employing effective excise taxes on tobacco, alcohol, and sugary beverages. https://www.bbhub.io/dotorg/sites/2/2019/04/Health-Taxes-to-Save-Lives.pdf. Accessed on April 14, 2021.

[88] Khanna M *et al.* 2021. Decentralized facility financing versus performance-based payments in primary health care: A large-scale randomized controlled trial in Nigeria. BMC Medicine. https://bmcmedicine.biomedcentral.com/articles/10.1186/s12916-021-02092-4. Accessed on September 24, 2021.

Chapter 8

Real-World Dynamics of Development Assistance for Health

"Doing less harm would be a good start. Beyond cutting back on aid, there are several other bad things that we could stop doing, and several good things that we should think about doing."

—Angus Deaton[a]

"Teacher don't teach me nonsense."

—Fela Anikulapo-Kuti[b]

Synopsis

Development Assistance for Health (DAH) is premised on a net flow of knowledge, know-how, and financial resources from the Global North to the Global South. Implicit in that construct are assumptions of a net superiority of the Global North in the production of better health for the Global South. Those assumptions have damaging implications in practice. The dynamics play out through multiple transactions and bargaining among the centers of influence, power, and perceived powerlessness in

---

[a]Deaton A. 2013. *The Great Escape: Health, Wealth, and the Origins of Inequality.* Princeton: Princeton University Press. p. 318.

[b]Anikulapo-Kuti F. Teacher don't teach me nonsense. https://felakuti.bandcamp.com/album/teacher-dont-teach-me-nonsense-1980. Accessed on May 28, 2021.

global health. There is much that is positive in DAH. However, there are vast areas of dysfunction, including the absurdity of self-serving announceables by powerful entities in the Global North, and devotion to fads that are presumed to be magic solutions to complex problems. The prevailing practice in much of the Global South fosters neo-dependency on the Global North; this is contrary to increasingly trendy notions that the problem of global health is that of neo-colonialism. There is a pressing need to do better. A break from ossified narratives and practices of DAH is central to such improvements.

8.1. The Premise of Development Assistance for Health

The practice of DAH is based on the proposition that a net flow of money, knowledge, and know-how from financiers (typically in the Global North) to recipients (typically in the Global South) will result in a net gain in health, health institutions, and health systems of recipient countries. The WHO reported that in 2017, external funding for health amounted to US\$16 billion. That was 0.2% of global health spending. Several key points stood out:[1]

- In the growing global economy that preceded the COVID-19 pandemic, donor financing fell from a high of US\$18 billion in 2014 to US\$16 billion in 2017. It declined in per capita US\$ and markedly as a proportion of Total Health Expenditures in LICs and LMICs since 2014.
- Despite that decline, donor funding for health remained important in many LICs and LMICs. At least 140 countries received external funding for health in 2017.
- In 2017, aid represented 29% of the health spending in LICs and 12% in LMICs. For 26 LICs and LMICs, of which 20 are in Sub-Saharan Africa, the level of reliance on donor funding is such that it constitutes more than 20% of their health spending.

Much has been written and continues to be written about the volume, trends, and potential trajectory of DAH. The major concerns and propositions include: how to finance the achievement of health dimensions of the

Sustainable Development Goals (SDGs);[2] characterizations of the past, present, and predicted future of global health spending;[3] estimation of spending to achieve progress in financing the priority areas of SDG3, the association between financing and outcomes, and identification of where resource gains are most needed;[4,5] levels of effort across donor countries;[6] measures of aid effectiveness,[7] DAH as an investment in health security;[8] and forms of catastrophic insurance against pandemics.[9]

One important strand of work, supported in part by WHO, has categorized DAH by function and has dual relevance to this chapter. First, it classified DAH into two parts: global (consisting of the supply of global public goods, management of cross-border externalities, and leadership and stewardship); and country specific (covering the provision of country-specific support to LICs, LMICs, and UMICs).[10] This is useful for clarifying where policy attention and scarce resources are best deployed over specified time periods. Second, it provides information on how global financiers reacted to the 2014–2015 Ebola epidemic in West Africa. In sum, between 2013 and 2015, international financing for global functions rose by US$1.4 billion to a total of US$7.3 billion. That increase was followed by a decline to US$7.0 billion in 2017. (The 2017 financing was about 24% of the total for ODA+, defined as such by the authors because it extends beyond the support typically reported in the International Development Statistics Database of the OECD's Development Assistance Committee to include public spending for pharmaceutical research and development for neglected diseases.)[11] Might the same trajectory be seen with the COVID-19 pandemic? In Chapter 9, we turn to a discussion of DAH for routine inputs to country-level health systems versus aid to support the provision of regional and global public goods.

The concerns and propositions noted above are in the context of long-running considerations of harmonization and alignment of DAH,[12] as detailed with much fanfare in the Paris Declaration on Aid Effectiveness, which, beyond its principles on effective aid, laid out a roadmap with lofty ambitions to improve by 2010 both the quality of aid and its development.[13] But how are they working out? The Quality of Official Development Assistance (QuODA) measures and compares providers of official development assistance (ODA) on quantitative indicators that matter most to development effectiveness and quality. It aims to encourage improvements to the quality of ODA by highlighting and assessing providers' performance. In the 2021 edition of QuODA, the largest *absolute* providers of aid — the United States, Germany, and the United Kingdom — ranked 35th, 28th, and 16th, respectively. Multilaterals dominated the overall rankings, taking each of the top five positions.[14]

This chapter is about the real-world interactions that determine and influence the level, scale, scope, and choices made with DAH. It covers the engagement between financiers on the one hand, and recipients on the other. It also provides insight into interactions among financiers. All these lead to the question of how DAH could be made more relevant to the realities of recipient countries, and how both recipients and financiers could do better to achieve two lofty goals: shifting from DAH that adds little value to DAH that adds higher value, and more rapid transition of countries out of recipient status. The question takes on new urgency in the context of the dual health and fiscal shocks caused by COVID-19.

8.2. Centers of Power, Influence, and Perceived Powerlessness

Much of the dynamics of DAH is about power and influence. Power, in this context, means the willingness and ability to set the terms of engagement by and with other players. This is done via the specification of goals and the shaping of the vocabulary of discourse among participants. The main categories of players are as follows:

- Country governments and regional/sub-regional intergovernmental institutions of the Global South.
- Multilateral financiers, including development banks and other global or regional multilateral financiers.
- Foundations.
- Government-funded bilateral agencies, including entities like JICA, SIDA, USAID, and disease-specific programs such as the United States President's Emergency Plan for AIDS Relief (PEPFAR) and the United States President's Malaria Initiative (US-PMI).
- Government funded-bilateral entities embedded within departments of trade.

- Product Development Partnerships, including research and development.
- Specialized Agencies (mostly of the United Nations), including variations of normative, technical, coordinating, convening, and some operational functions.
- Think tanks.
- NGOs originating from the Global South.
- NGOs originating from the Global North.
- Private sector contractors who deliver services funded by DAH.
- High-net-worth individuals.
- Celebrity figures in the arts, entertainment, and sports.

Each category of actors in global health includes members with at least some functional capacity to exercise power in DAH, but relatively few recognize, choose to, and have the effective capacity to exercise the power. Just as the exercise of power can be learned, powerlessness can be learned and become a habit. The evolution of DAH — over the past three decades, at least — is such that the current construct of power and who most exercises it has become baked into the network of participants. That recognition of how things have been is different from acceptance that it is the way things should be and could be, as manifested by the contemporary discourse on the colonial or quasicolonial origins of global health,[15] and on the importance of "decolonizing" global health and the framing of discourse about it. I will return to the matter of decolonization later in this chapter.

Those with the most direct access to powerful individuals and institutions have considerable opportunities to influence the terms of engagement in DAH, even though they might not be the sole or dominant deciders in a particular situation.

Taken in isolation, each category of players makes sense, albeit to different degrees. When multiplied by the number of programs, the landscape becomes very unwieldy, a situation that is compounded by the seemingly perpetual lives of many of the organizations and their propensity for mission creep. A few examples will suffice. The real and perceived inadequacies of WHO's response to the HIV/AIDS pandemic, especially after the demise of its Special Program on AIDS (renamed the Global

Program on AIDS), laid the basis for establishing the Joint United Nations Program on HIV/AIDS (UNAIDS) in 1994. Twenty-seven years later, the rationale for the continued existence of UNAIDS as a distinct program is very tenuous. The GFATM was created largely in response to the perceived and real inadequacies in the levels of funding that pre-GFATM financiers of development assistance — like the World Bank — brought to the control of HIV/AIDS, TB, and malaria. The GFATM, like Gavi, has since ventured into financing health systems strengthening, with no strong empirical evidence of its fitness for purpose and impact in that domain. PEPFAR brought enormous resources to the HIV/AIDS response and it expanded access to key technologies for infection prevention and treatment. It also struggles with questions about country-owned financial sustainability and the program's unintended distortionary effects on health financing, ownership, and the architecture of service delivery within countries.

Compounding the above is the pervasive attention-deficit hyperactivity disorder (ADHD) in much of global health. Eradication campaigns give way to control and elimination programs, then eradication comes back on the agenda with sudden outbreaks of enthusiasm. Off-budget foreign aid gives way to mixtures of budget support and sector program financing, then it swings back to off-budget support. United Nations agencies like WHO come with the political legitimacy of the United Nations, but they also come with its sluggishness, which partly explains the allure of parallel or competing entities that are nimbler, and whose policies are more directly susceptible to the actionable whims of their largest financiers.

WHO ought to function as the north star in global health, but it is suffering from an acute-on-chronic form of ADHD. WHO gets its funding from two main sources: assessed contributions from Member States and voluntary contributions from Member States and other partners. Assessed contributions are a percentage of a country's GDP as agreed by the UN General Assembly, and they cover less than 20% of WHO's total budget.[16] The remainder of WHO's financing comes from voluntary contributions made by Member States, other UN agencies, intergovernmental organizations, philanthropic foundations, the private sector, and other sources. Thus, 80% of WHO is purchasable by special interests and WHO has become a *de-facto* general contractor to financiers of programs funded outside the budget raised from assessed contributions. The global health compass is dysfunctional, fluttering, and oscillating across the spectrum of uncritical cheerleaders at one extreme, a group that supports it without undue coddling in the middle, and those who use it as a whipping child at the other extreme. Most importantly, WHO conflates a broad mandate with an infinite capacity to know and do everything well. This situation portrays a lack of institutional discipline to recognize the importance of prioritization, embrace the reality of trade-offs, and deploy its comparative advantages.

The landscape of DAH is now a network of the groups of actors listed above. The dynamics among them vary with time, place, and purpose. They function as individual entities, as partners, as collaborating competitors, and as competing collaborators in a global theater.

8.3. Substance, Theater, and Announceables

As global health has become a common feature on the agendas of the G7 and G20 groups of nations, so has it become a tool for statecraft and stagecraft. Sometimes, it is deployed in a manner that drives home a specific policy objective and clarifies choices at the highest levels of international discourse. An example of this is the short piece by Japan's Deputy Prime Minister and Finance Minister Taro Aso on the role of Ministries of Finance in achieving UHC: first, seek to achieve UHC early in the development process; second, use domestic resources to finance UHC; third, use external resources to complement domestic funding of UHC; and fourth, address the financial challenges of a rapidly aging population.[17] His commentary reflected Japan's agenda-setting role within the G7, which was captured in the Kobe Communiqué G7 Health Ministers' Meeting of September 2016.[18]

Another example of mindset-shifting leadership is that shown by South African President Cyril Ramaphosa on COVID-19, both on prevention and in an African strategy for vaccines.[19] Ramaphosa's leadership marked a decisive shift from continental dependency on the timeline of any single source to a portfolio approach. Ramaphosa, in his capacity as Chair of the AU, established the COVID-19 African Vaccine Acquisition

Task Team (AVATT) as a component to support the Africa Vaccine Strategy that was endorsed by the AU Bureau of Heads of State and Government in August 2020.

Institutional powers can drive positive change, and such changes abound in global health. Three of the most remarkable involved the WHO's leadership of three programs: the eradication of smallpox;[20] the Onchocerciasis Control Program and the African Program for Onchocerciasis Control;[21,22] and the Framework Convention on Tobacco Control.[23]

These examples of the use of political power to drive substantive agendas, in varying combinations of North–South engagement, indicate what is possible in a positive sense. On the other hand, there abound many instances of sheer vanity in global health, leading to a waste of time and consuming energies that could have been put to productive use elsewhere. Composite Vignette 8.1 illustrates an elaborate exercise that consumed the time and collective brain space of many across the Global North and the Global South, with no discernible benefit to the health of the Global South.

Composite Vignette 8.1. Distortionary Use of Announceables

George D. Parsons, an unknown on the global stage, had just come into office as Head of Government in the Republic of Suprema, a G7 country. Seeking to establish his cachet as a player on the global stage, his advisers came up with the idea of establishing a Global Coalition for Health (GCH). Even some of those advisers had qualms about this move, as there were plenty of global coalitions for various dimensions of health, and it was not clear what value this one would add. Eventually, the allure of an announceable outweighed all other considerations. Then Laurel Jacobs, Head of Global Health in Suprema's Foreign Aid Ministry, called Jan van Kindermans, Vice-President for Health at the Global Monetary Institute (GMI); the Head of Government needed an announceable, pursuant to which his Government would spearhead a new Global Coalition for Health. Kindermans sighed and made some noises about complicating an already crowded coordination landscape in Global Health. Jacobs, usually mild mannered, dismissed the protestations and reminded Kindermans of the

(Continued)

Composite Vignette 8.1. (*Continued*)

forthcoming round of financing for GMI, to which Suprema's contribution would be key. Kindermans made a swift decision; this was not something on which he would spend his social capital with his Director General, who would surely be informed if he declined. The Director-General's term was up for extension and this was no time to irritate Suprema.

The machinery of GMI sprang into action. In a cynical mockery of a country-led global exercise, Kindermans instructed his team to reach out to Ministers of Health across LICs and MICs in Africa, Asia, Latin America and the Caribbean, and the Middle East. Those ministers were to ask GMI to co-convene, with the Government of Suprema, a new mechanism, the GCH, to help solve all their health systems' problems. Nobody had reason to believe that the new GCH was substantively different from the myriad of such mechanisms already established. The GCH was announced with much fanfare: press releases with turgid quotes and lofty claims, and praise for the wisdom of the new leader, whose commitment would lead the world to great things.

There followed series upon series of meetings to define the vision, mission, goals, and objectives of GCH. Sensing the possibility of some grant financing, multiple agencies argued over who would head which aspect of the GCH and who would host its secretariat. Failing to reach agreement on the latter, they decided to have three co-hosts; GCH would have its secretariat in three different agencies on three different continents. Since each agency held that its mandate was the most important of all, GCH had as many "priorities" as it had members. Its funding plan was an incoherent assemblage of special interest pleading. The meetings continued, and so did the colorful statements about coordination of coordinators. The Ministers of Health from LICs and MICs had seen similar theater before and were not surprised.

Institutional envy and the fear of missing out are strong motivators on the global stage. Three other G7 countries demanded a piece of the action; the heads of their foreign-aid agencies came under pressure from their political leaders to justify their own lack of press coverage. Why should the new leader of Suprema have all the fun and glory? The three cosecretariats knew they had a problem, and they came up with an ingenious plan. The solution, they thought, was an Enhanced GCH (E-GCH), but that did not satisfy the other three G7 leaders, who insisted on having clear markers of

(Continued)

Composite Vignette 8.1. (*Continued*)

their own priorities. The solution was to add a "plus" for each of the three G7 countries, and thus was born the GCH+++. Now everyone could lay claim to the GCH.

The substance-free hype continued for years in the form of meetings with no decisions other than to hold follow-up meetings. Any associated pledge of financing was a magical reshuffling of prior allocations and unfulfilled pledges.

Ten years after its launch, there was no verifiable evidence that the GCH+++ had added any value to the work of countries. There was no evaluation of its work. That seemed to be the basis for declaring it a success. With much fanfare, the GCH+++ was repurposed to serve as the coordinating mechanism that would lead countries to achieve Health for All by the Year 2050. It was yet another announceable.

8.4. The Eternal Search for Universal Solutions

Few things in global health are more wasteful than debates about vertical versus diagonal versus horizontal or integrated approaches to investing in health. Yet, those debates endure even at the highest levels, despite the very mixed empirical evidence on the integration of targeted interventions and health systems.[24] The debates typically run as binary portrayals of integrated (horizontal) versus nonintegrated (vertical) programs and are characterized by polarized views. Protagonists for and against argue the relative merits and demerits of each approach.

The presence of both integrated and nonintegrated programs in many countries suggests benefits — and likely problems — to each approach,[25] but the discourse has persisted beyond the post-Alma Ata duel between proponents of comprehensive primary health care and proponents of selective primary health care, which Professor Kenneth Newell memorably called a counter-revolution.[26] Perhaps the allure of finding the one approach that will always work has special mystique in a field that is very complex, subject to socio-political narratives, and fraught with emergent dynamics in multiple systems that defy universal prescriptions.

Perhaps the desire for headline-grabbing success stories creates fertile grounds for trite approaches couched in gobbledygook that has the blessing of the collective. Perhaps the rarity of rigorously evaluated successes drives perceived needs for single-country success stories that could be used to justify the preferences of donors, regardless of inattention to the "compared to what?" question.

There are legitimate issues of vertical programs distorting national priorities and programs,[27,28] but the counterfactual in many LICs and LMICs, in practice, is generally not an effective system that steadily improves health outcome. Might those much-vilified vertical programs be distorting a long-standing *status quo* of harmonious mediocrity? One source of angst is the question of where the money goes, with worries that investments in systems have not been as well funded as those in vertical programs.[29] An implicit assumption is that the opportunity cost of investing in a vertical program is an investment in health system strengthening, which is inherently good until proven otherwise. Yet, there is little or no empirical evidence to justify this assumption.[30] All these raise questions about the mission creep of agencies such as the GFATM and Gavi to establish Health Systems Windows or Business Lines. WHO's remarkably named publication, entitled "Everybody's Business,"[31] unwittingly signalled a lack of awareness that not every institution or individual has a comparative advantage in health systems.

A close look at the financing of health system development in Bangladesh reveals some of the challenges. Bangladesh offers many lessons because of the duration of multidonor collaboration with its government in the joint financing of agreed work programs, the sheer size of the country and the programs, and the complex interplay of government, domestic NGOs, and international actors. The program data here are from the Implementation Completion Review of the Health Sector Development Program in Bangladesh,[32] unless specified otherwise.

The objective of the Health Sector Development Program in Bangladesh, which lasted from 2011 to 2017, was "to enable the Recipient to strengthen health systems and improve health services, particularly for the poor." The objective did not change during implementation. Additional financing was provided together with some restructuring of the project in 2016, which included adjustment of some outcome targets for improvement in health services. The Program was structured to be implemented as a sector-wide approach (SWAp), financing a specific slice of the national Health, Population, and Nutrition Sector Development Program (HPNSDP). The total estimated cost of the HPNSDP at project appraisal was US$8,011 million, of which the government was expected to provide US$5,844 million and external financiers or development partners (DPs) US$2,167 million.

At appraisal, Australian Aid, CIDA, UK DFID, the European Commission, the KfW, GIZ, JICA, Swedish International Development Cooperation Agency (Sida), UNFPA, UNAIDS, UNICEF, World Bank (IDA), WHO, and USAID had expressed indicative commitment for a total of US$1,606.24 million. USAID was the largest development partner, providing US$450 million to HPNSDP (20.8% of external financing). The World Bank was the second largest development partner, contributing, at appraisal, US$358.9 million in IDA financing (16.6% of external financing).

The World Bank provided fiduciary and technical oversight to DP contributions through multi- and single-donor trust funds (US$365 million in total), building on the experience of the previous health SWAp implemented in Bangladesh. The World Bank approved US$ 150 million of additional financing in June 2016, to fill a financing gap in the last year of project implementation, bringing the total World Bank IDA commitment to US$508 million. At appraisal, 70% of the project funds were to be spent under Component 1 (Improving Service Delivery) and 30% under Component 2 (Strengthening Health Systems). The final distribution of spending by component (which included the US$150 million of the additional financing) showed a relative increase under Component 2 (from 30% to 43%) and decrease under Component 1 (from 70% to 57%) (Table 8.1). Among the key lessons were the following:

- **Managing pooled funds for health:** In large programs, with multiple pooling partners, effective coordination and consultation mechanisms among the Bank, DPs, and government are essential to avoid fragmentation/duplication of efforts, reduce transaction costs, and align project objectives to a country's development needs. The Project enhanced coordination and consultation mechanisms among DPs by

Table 8.1.   Rating the Health Sector Development Program in Bangladesh

Parameter	Description	"Efficacy" Rating (Achievement of Objectives)
Objective 1	Strengthen health systems	Modest
Objective 2 (Original)	Improve health services, particularly for the poor (original outcome targets)	Substantial
Objective 2 (Revised)	Improve health services, particularly for the poor (revised outcome targets)	High
Overall	Combined	Substantial

Source: Adapted from IEG Review Team. 2018. *Bangladesh — BD: Health Sector Development Program (English)*. Washington, D.C.: World Bank Group. https://documents.worldbank.org/en/publication/documents-reports/documentdetail/114181528922648368/bangladesh-bd-health-sector-development-program. Accessed on March 11, 2021.

conducting joint missions and providing coordinated technical assistance with different partners leading different themes. The establishment of the Local Consultative Group on Health also improved coordination and harmonization of DP's support.

- **Disbursement-Linked Indicators and Incentive Structures:** Effectiveness of the disbursement-linked-indicator (DLI) approach is attenuated when budgetary incentives are only partly associated with the achievement of results. In this project, the government budget for the HPNSDP was prefinanced by the Ministry of Finance at the beginning of each fiscal year, which reduced the effectiveness of the incentive structure of a project with DLIs.

The program in Bangladesh was implicitly a flagship[33] of an approach to reduce the fragmentation of financing that is appropriately decried by many parties and a rationale for the search for harmonization and alignment across governments and external financiers.[34,35] It also indicates the challenges of any single magic formula. On the one hand, Program "efficacy" was judged as "substantial" in improving health services, particularly for the poor. On the other hand, it was rated "modest" in strengthening health systems — in precisely the domain of work that is supposed to be the principal attraction of SWAp-type investments. The finding in Bangladesh was not rare for sector support operations, considering experiences elsewhere.

In the 1990s, there was much prospective hype over the Zambia Health Sector Support Project. Yet, according to the project Implementation Completion Report:[36]

> *"There is no evidence to suggest that the project had any measurable impact on the health status of the Zambian population. It is also difficult to ascribe to it significant improvements in the functioning of the health system, which was its main objective. The project did help to sustain district-level health care through purchases of equipment, drugs and medicines. However, it did not adequately address capacity weaknesses in the health sector, and its investments in civil works were not considered to be cost effective. The external monitoring and evaluation (M&E) component was inadequate to the extent that information on the project's impact was not available at the time of completion. Credit must be given to the project team for its substantial contributions to the policy dialogue on (i) decentralization, (ii) financing reforms and (iii) proposed separation of financing from the provision of services under the Government of Zambia's (GRZ) health reform program. By contrast, the actual contribution from project investments toward these achievements is debatable."*

The experience in Ghana is more nuanced and equally instructive. The Ghana Health Sector Support project involved the government and a broad swathe of international development and financing institutions. The external cofinanciers in a pooled funding approach were DANIDA, DFID, the Netherlands, Nordic Fund, and the World Bank. According to the Implementation Completion Report Review,[37] the objective was to support the Government's reform of the health sector through implementation of its Medium-Term Health Strategy, and the project was handled under an instrument that was new at the time, a SWAp. There were no preidentified components. Noteworthy aspects of the outcomes included the following, according to the same Implementation Completion Report Review:

- Sector-wide policy changes were introduced because of the overall project. Funding, training, and equipment helped to strengthen decentralization of decision making to regional and district management teams. There was no significant progress in improving intersectoral collaboration by the health sector, or collaboration with the private sector.

- Some health outputs improved. However, persistent regional inequalities in access to services continued, and many infectious disease programs failed to meet their targets. (For example, the TB detection target rate was 85% but reached 45%; for malaria, 40% of children under 5 were to be sleeping under impregnated bed nets but only 9% were reached; and the number of Guinea Worm cases increased.)

- Certain shortcomings were highlighted. A comprehensive human resource strategy was not developed for the sector as a whole and persistent regional inequality in access to services continued. Overall utilization of public health services remained low. High rates of manpower turnover at the central level had weakened institutional memory, which might affect project sustainability. Except for the initial core donor group, all other donors remained outside of the resource pooling system, and some participating donors were maintaining earmarked funding which reduces the benefits of shared funding. Progress in the integration of private providers in planning and service delivery was far slower than intended; and contracts to regulate the collaboration between the public and not-for-profit private sectors were still to be developed. Intersectoral collaboration remained weak; no guidelines, policies or mechanisms were instituted to make the health sector work more effectively with other sectors (i.e., with nutrition, sanitation, education, agriculture, and social welfare). Monitorable indicators to cover inputs, outputs, and outcomes should have been developed at the design stage of the project, rather than relying on data from the Demographic and Health Surveys, which were not tailored to the project issues nor the project schedule.

The Second Health Sector Program Support Project provides even more insight, based on the Implementation Completion Report Review.[38] Noteworthy aspects of the outcomes included the following:

- The overall outcome rating was Moderately Unsatisfactory. Access to services, quality, financing, partnerships, and health financing were all rated as "Modest." Project Efficiency was rated as "Negligible."

- On health outcomes, the report noted that between 1998 and 2003, there were no improvements in child health outcomes. Likewise, there was no statistically significant change in total fertility (4.6 in 1998 and 4.4 in 2003). Ghana Health Services Data on malnutrition revealed no major trends of improvement.
- On dealing with development partners, the review found some clear successes in working through common management arrangements and continuing the policy and planning dialogue of the SWAp. Yet, some development partners increasingly moved toward project management support with earmarked funding, including off-budget financing, undermining the effectiveness of the SWAp partnership. Private sector facilities were still not included during health sector planning or budgeting, and they were not included in monitoring progress in the sector.

The three cases explored above do not constitute proof of the usefulness or otherwise of SWAps. However, they suggest serious issues that should be addressed instead of finessed, glossed over, or ignored. There is no multicountry empirical evidence that the SWAp approach results in a net reduction of transaction costs of coordination. Do they really reduce transaction costs, or do they merely change the nature of transactions from multiple and separate lines of communication between each financier and the government, to multiple, overly ponderous series of meetings within the groups of donors, and then between the donors and governments?

The political drive and the cult-like proselytism around SWAps far outweighed the objectively verifiable evidence of their net effects on strengthening health systems, reducing transaction costs, and improving health outcomes when compared to other approaches. Have the countries traded the problems of multiple, time-consuming bilateral negotiations with individual donors for a construct in which groups of donors form a cartel to gang up against the country's Ministry of Health, wasting a lot of time on review meetings about processes without attention to substance?

The point here is not an argument for or against any particular approach. It is a call for clarity around four questions:

(a) What are the country and the financiers optimizing for?

(b) In each context, what is the most appropriate approach or combination of approaches and instruments to reach those goals?

(c) How and to whom are external financiers held accountable?

(d) How will success be measured, and compared to what?

Attention to these three questions would minimize the risk of a mismatch between ends and means. Most importantly, it would minimize risks of irrationally escalating commitments to any single approach of dubious empirical value.

8.5. From Neo-colonialism to Neo-dependency

There is much contemporary commentary on the malaise of colonization, for its historical significance and for its contemporary resonance in global health.[39–47] The proposition that global health retains and thrives on its roots in colonial adventures has merit. Egregious imbalances persist in the power dynamics between the Global North and the Global South. Technical assistance mostly means Northerners, with *presumed* expertise and cringeworthy condescension, telling Southerners what to do.

The presumption of expertise is important. In my experience, while many from the Global North have deep subject matter expertise, work hard to truly understand the realities of their clients and counterparts, and make serious effort to enable the success of their clients and host countries, many others are mediocre at best, and many are shockingly unqualified. The mediocre and the unqualified thrive on an implicit benefit of the doubt that merely being from the Global North means the individual has any expertise worth sharing. That benefit of the doubt is rarely accorded their peers from the Global South, even when the latter not only have similar professional preparation, but often have superior professional preparation and deeper understanding of the operational context. Some cases would be laughable if they were not tragic. It is possible for a character from the Global North, with nothing more than an undergraduate education in general theology, to self-parade and hold sway in powerful groups as a guru in global health, to pontificate on epidemiology, malariology, health economics, policies, and strategies, and to seek to lecture those who know better just because those being lectured are from the

Global South. This absurdity has become entrenched as an incestuous network of mediocre good old boys and good old girls from the Global North.

Yet another dimension of neo-colonialism in global health is the inability or refusal of some from the Global North to read the room. I have seen many galling examples of this problem. One of the most memorable in Kinshasa was that of a Belgian lecturing a room that included eye-rolling Congolese officials on the importance of human rights and accountability. One wondered whether this Belgian studied so little history that he was oblivious to a central dynamic at play: direct or indirect beneficiaries of organized plunder, terror, and historical crimes against humanity in the Congo[48,49] ought to do more listening than lecturing about human rights and accountability in that part of the world.

Those from the Global North who are least qualified are often the same ones who portray a sense of entitlement to tell the Global South what to do. I witnessed an occasion during which the Minister of Health of a recipient country in Central and Eastern Europe stated that he was agnostic about which consultant worked with his team, provided that they met his specified qualifications. The lead representative of the bilateral donor protested mightily, claiming to know what was best. This was strange, considering that the consultant was going to do the development equivalent of surgery on the minister's country. If a patient went for surgery and insisted that the surgeon provide proof of certification by the College of Surgeons, surely that would be a reasonable request?

In another country in the WHO's Eastern Mediterranean Region, in 2015 a colleague and I got a sad story from a senior country official who had been at the receiving end of shoddy technical assistance that had been funded by yet another bilateral financier. The contractor's assignment was to develop a computer-enabled management system for a major hospital, with the clear duty to ensure the transfer of skills to host country nationals. But, according to the country official, the contracted firm simply did the day-to-day work by itself and nothing on capacity building. About six months before the end of the multi-year contract, the contractor reportedly told the country official that if the firm left on schedule, the system would collapse because the local team would not be able to run it. The contractor then told the country official to ask the bilateral funding agency, which had hired the contractor, to extend the contract in order to avoid that collapse.

Each of the examples above might have qualified for inclusion in the book entitled *Annoying: The Science of What Bugs Us*.[50] But the challenge goes beyond some bad apples — or bad mangoes, since these acts do occur in warmer climates too. They are more fundamental than mere annoyance. Indeed, they are manifestations of an ecosystem that permits egregious levels of rent seeking, charlatanism, and predatory behavior by unscrupulous purveyors of DAH-funded technical assistance. They are the more visible tentacles of neo-colonization. Picture a head of a Northern NGO who promised to champion with a G7 government the replenishment effort of an international institution. That sounded like an altruistic move until it became clear that there was the expectation of a quid-pro-quo. The would-be champion, who used to work in the front office of a head of government, sought a strategic partnership with that institution to give the NGO the kind of access and policy leverage that no NGO from Nepal, Nicaragua, or Niger could have. Fueled by the Global North's legacy of smug entitlement, such rapacious rent seeking and policy capture are common in global health.

In 2015, a crusading Northerner went to Sierra Leone during the Ebola outbreak and made lofty promises to doctors and nurses in one of the hospitals. A few years later, those health workers told one of my colleagues and me that they had heard nothing from the would-be savior. It was harrowing to hear their narrative of being used as props for photo opportunities in yet another round of global health ethno-tourism.

A final example of inappropriate technical assistance is behavioral, in the form of the all-knowing "experts" from the Global North who just will not listen to *the natives*. They must speak all the time, talk over country officials, and have determined the conclusion before the forum started. *Whether one believes in evolution or creation, I suppose there is a reason that humans have one mouth that can close and two ears that are always open: in most situations, it is prudent to do twice as much listening as talking.* Why can't these "experts" from the Global North practice this art? It is because of a sense of entitlement that often manifests as hubris — and yet another derivative of neo-colonization.

Despite the above, there are serious flaws in the current flurry of calls to decolonize global health. The most serious flaw is the inattention to *neo-dependency*, which is a clear and growing danger to the already tenuous accountability of many Global South governments to their own populations for policies, programs, and health outcomes. The clamor for decolonization unwittingly presumes that the burden of changing the terms of engagement falls on colonizers of the past and dominant Global North powers of the present. While that might be attractive in purely academic terms or the wishful thinking of reflex activism on social media, it will achieve neither *fundamental* effectiveness nor *durable* traction in practice. Without a credible economic or geopolitical threat, the colonizer has no incentive to voluntarily give up advantages that come from the *status quo*. Plaintive calls for decolonization will not produce change. The colonized must self-emancipate, absent which calls for decolonization will be no more durable than transient analgesia of the colonized.

Yet another flaw of the decolonization emphasis is a failure to recognize that the Global South has not gained respect because donors from the Global North are all too aware of the brazen corruption and looting of public funds by politicians and office holders in the Global South, who stash looted funds in London, New York, Paris, and Zurich. The replenishment sessions of some global financiers, with enablers from the Global South holding their proverbial begging bowls, come across as internet-enabled minstrel shows. Public figures from the Global South show up at pledging sessions, begging for money to save lives in their countries — in cahoots with Northern performative activists, academics who would magically eradicate poverty by turning the treasuries of the Global North over to the Global South, and faded-popstars-turned-saviors of the photogenic poor. These theaters of absurdity enable self-adulating operators from the Global North to use many from the Global South as props and claques. To paraphrase the late Professor Chinua Achebe, narcissistic charity is the opium of Northern saviors. Professor Oyewale Tomori, an eminent virologist and former member of the Gavi Board, put it this way:

"GAVI has done a great job, but it has also hampered development in recipient countries. The last question I asked at a GAVI meeting was 'Is GAVI forever?' And my reason for asking was that so many African governments — even when their economies are developed enough — revert to GAVI-assistance instead of taking care of their own people."[51]

Beyond the supplicant's narrative of decolonization, a far more robust proposition is that countries of the Global South should take responsibility to stop the practice of depending upon the Global North for their own core policy priority setting processes and for financing their most basic health system functions and health care delivery. Doing so is essential but will not be easy for many countries that have normalized neo-dependency, as illustrated in Composite Vignette 8.2.

Composite Vignette 8.2. Culpable Neo-dependency

Dr. Afua Ngugi-Traore sighed. It had been a long week. It started with a query from The Daily Observer, whose reporter harangued her about user fees for health services at the Regional Health Department where Dr. Ngugi-Traore was Director and Chief Medical Officer (D-CMO). A Europe-based NGO, whose name translated into "Free Health for All," had informed the reporter about user fees at the District Hospital. Then all hell broke loose after the paper published the reporter's interview with Dr. Ngugi-Traore, who specifically requested to go on the record and on camera. She told the reporter that she was sick and tired of being blamed for doing what was needed to keep the hospital running amidst the "incompetence and hypocrisy" of senior officials from the Republic of Ryagua's Ministry of Health, Health Insurance Agency, and Ministry of Finance, as well as "clueless NGOs from Europe." Two days after the TV interview, the Minister of Health sacked Dr. Ngugi-Traore for "insubordination and conduct that is contrary to civil service norms."

Someone at HealthWatch tipped off the Universal Broadcasting Service, whose journalists contacted Dr. Ngugi-Traore to request her appearance on Blunt Talk, a highly rated television program that is watched by millions of people across the world.

(Continued)

Composite Vignette 8.2. (*Continued*)

Blunt Talk: Dr. Ngugi-Traore, welcome to Blunt Talk, where we hold nothing back.

Dr. Ngugi-Traore: Thank you for having me on your show.

Blunt Talk: Let's get to the point. You accused multiple government departments of incompetence and hypocrisy without a shred of evidence. Why?

Dr. Ngugi-Traore: There is plenty of evidence. In addition to being incompetent and hypocritical, they are also irresponsible. Let me give you a summary, then we can go into details as you wish. Our country has seen some economic growth. We have no great oil wealth, so our economy thrives on the service industry, the nascent manufacturing capacity, agriculture, and the small but growing tourism. In short, we depend on the brains and brawns of our people. But the government is ignoring their health, the very health needed to build human capital.

Blunt Talk: How so?

Dr. Ngugi-Traore: It is the case that Ryagua is now a middle-income country and expected to graduate or transition out of grant-based foreign aid. Soon, we will be eligible for only loans; no more grants, and little if any concessional credits.

Blunt Talk: That is something to be proud of, isn't it?

Dr. Ngugi-Traore: Normally, yes. But there is a failure to graduate. Or a refusal to graduate. The Ministry of Finance and the Ministry of Health have taken no action to make up for the loss of funds that will happen when the country graduates from its dependency on foreign aid for basic health services. We are already seeing the effects in terms of reduced funds for health services. Across my region, hospitals are experiencing worsening shortages of basic supplies, diagnostics, and medicines. Our health centers will soon lack basic vaccines.

Blunt Talk: Surely the ministers must be aware of that?

Dr. Ngugi-Traore: They are all too aware of it. The problem is their reaction. When my fellow D-CMOs and I asked them about it during our annual forum, they told us to calm down. Their calculus is that all Ryagua has to do is nothing. Then those foreigners who love us more than we love ourselves will proclaim emergencies, raise money during pledging sessions on CNN, BBC, and France 24, and the grant-financed programs will continue to be funded somehow. It is a very cozy arrangement for all the parties.

(Continued)

Composite Vignette 8.2. (*Continued*)

Blunt Talk: Really?

Dr. Ngugi-Traore: Really.

Blunt Talk: But what about your hospitals and health centers. How are you managing?

Dr. Ngugi-Traore: Let me help you rephrase that. It should be how I was managing, since I am no longer on duty in the region.

Blunt Talk: My mistake. Please continue.

Dr. Ngugi-Traore: We had two choices. The first was to stop admitting patients because we had no funds to run the hospital. The other was to continue admitting them, but to charge them user fees, even though we hated doing so, seeing as many of them found it hard to pay the fees.

Blunt Talk: I see. But you never called it user fees in any official declaration.

Dr. Ngugi-Traore: We did not. We called the scheme "Shared Solidarity for Sustainability."

Blunt Talk: That sounds like Love Your Mother! Nobody would disagree with the principle.

Dr. Ngugi-Traore: Exactly right.

Blunt Talk: What do you say about the accusation made by "Free Health For All," that you imposed user fees as part of a neo-liberal plot favored by western interests?

Dr. Ngugi-Traore: That is utter nonsense. I'm sick and tired of clueless northern NGOs who act as if we cannot think for ourselves. It is a convenient and lazy trope that gets them headlines for their fundraising. User fees are bad in that they cause financial hardship for our people. The solution lies with our own government, which does not take seriously its own responsibilities, not with external agencies.

Blunt Talk: You have very strongly held views and claim the government's conduct is making the country an object of ridicule. How so?

Dr. Ngugi-Traore: Let me share a small example with you. Last year, I was invited to join the county's delegation to the Board meeting of the World Health Finance Consortium. The Minister made an impassioned plea during the plenary session for a grant to buy condoms for our country's HIV/AIDS Program. Then the Board took a lunch break. I was standing in line and overheard two famous delegates from donor countries discussing our Minister's pitch. According to one of them, "These people have no shame. They want us to give them our taxpayers' money so that they can have sex!"

(Continued)

Composite Vignette 8.2. (*Continued*)

Blunt Talk: Oh, dear. Do you have any final thoughts to share with our viewers?

Dr. Ngugi-Traore: It is fair and proper to condemn colonialism and its continuing effects on our country's health system. It is vital to condemn and reverse the culpable neo-dependency of our leaders and our country.

Blunt Talk: Thank you, Dr. Ngugi-Traore, for coming to Blunt Talk.

Dr. Ngugi-Traore: Thanks for having me on your show.

8.6. Partners and Derailers

In *Reforming the Unreformable*,[52] Ngozi Okonjo-Iweala notes that the international community can be a powerful ally to support reform in a developing country by speaking out or backing reforms. She also cautions that members of the international community can be fickle and play largely to their own interests, so reformers would be wise not to put too much stock in their goodwill and support. Those observations and cautionary notes apply to global health.

The international community has proven to be a force for good in many dimensions of global health and across every region of the world. Some of the actions are at the country level, while others are at the regional level. Contemporary examples of such engagement abound across policy analyses, convening, and financing in, among many others: Turkey's Health Transformation Program, which drove progress to Universal Health Coverage in that country;[53] the National treatment program of hepatitis C in Egypt;[54] Ethiopia's Health Extension Program;[55] Chile's Study of Hospital Concessions;[56] and China's quest for health sector transformation,[57] which was a collaboration among the Government of China, WHO, and the World Bank. Emphasis here is on the sense of purpose, a grounding in the legitimate policy direction of the country and its government, *de facto* duty of care, evidence of serious effort, and a commitment to learning instead of ex-ante declaration that any one path is the holy grail; if all are present, it would be unfair to blame the international community for program failures, since such failures could arise from factors outside the foreseeable control of any party.

The international community also demonstrates aversion to progress and to the empowerment of Southern institutions, especially when such empowerment comes at the expense of entrenched interests of institutions that are dominated by the Global North. Where major shifts in power or institutional functions are at stake, even mission-critical initiatives can be crippled or delayed by a combination of special interests, *status quo* bias, and confirmation bias as illustrated in Composite Vignette 8.3.

Composite Vignette 8.3. Ossified Mandates, Vanity Projects, and Turfism

Angela Coumba cut a weary figure as she boarded the plane at New York's JFK airport on her way back to her home country of Bumania on the continent of Kawanda. She had just had a brutally frank discussion with Jack Stevens, CEO of the World Development Fund. Coumba, a distinguished professor of epidemiology, former director of the Kawanda Health Consortium, and former United Nations Diplomat, had met with Stevens in one of the countless side meetings of the United Nations General Assembly (UNGA). Coumba and Stevens knew each other from their younger days as up-and-coming professionals, and theirs was a healthy relationship based on mutual respect. Until now.

In the wake of the devastating outbreak of Meloba Hemorrhagic Fever in West Kawanda in 2014–2016, Coumba had made a public case for more local, national, and regional investments in Kawanda's capacity for disease surveillance, detection, preparedness, and response. She expected Stevens to see the merit of the case. Stevens initially was evasive. When pressed, Stevens informed Coumba that he was acting on the advice of his Principal Economist for Kawanda, who vehemently asserted during the 2014–2016 Meloba outbreak that since most government health spending in Kawanda was not pro-poor, it would be wrong to invest more in health in Kawanda. This made no sense to Coumba, who reminded Stevens that Kawandan Union Heads of State had formally established the Kawanda Network for Disease Control and Prevention, with its hub in Binshasa. They were

(Continued)

Composite Vignette 8.3. (*Continued*)

making an effort and could use some help. Coumba always had a core of steel beneath her warm exterior. She pointedly wondered why Stevens, who ought to know better, was hiding behind nonsensical advice from people who had been described as "third-rate economists from first-rate universities."[58] She implored her old colleague to cut out the obfuscation and asked him what special interest was preventing him from doing what was so blindingly obvious.

Seeing that Coumba would not drop the case, Stevens convened a meeting of his peers across agencies in the margins of the 2019 UNGA in New York. By then, there had been several other epidemics in parts of Kawanda: Meloba in the center, yellow fever in the south, cholera in the west, and Hepatitis C in the north-east.

The meeting was a disaster of epic proportions. Stevens's Regional Adviser for Kawanda and his Chief Director for Health asserted that Kawanda would never have a viable regional network because Kawandans simply couldn't manage any regional enterprise. "They don't and will never have the capacity to run an agency." They cited the problems of the Kawandan Center for Capacity Building as proof. Coumba was appalled. She asked when the World Development Fund would advise the United States to dissolve all its institutions, given the dysfunction of its Congress, and when it would advise the European Union to do the same, given the mess of its bureaucracy and the dysfunction of the Euro, Brexit, and the Greek fiscal debacle.

Pauline Milla, the Regional Manager of the Alliance for Global Health, chimed in with the claim that there was no need for the Kawanda Network for Disease Control and Prevention, since such things were squarely within the mandate of the Alliance for Global Health. Stevens scoffed at that assertion, reminding the gathering that the Alliance for Global Health had bungled the response to the Meloba outbreak in West Kawanda in 2014–2016. "It takes a lot of chutzpah to claim that having failed at a subregional level, you must now permanently take charge at the regional level. You should find ways to collaborate with and not undermine the Kawanda Network for Disease Control and Prevention. That said, it won't work. The solution is the innovation that my Chief Health Director and I have started, the Pandemic Urgency Fund. It is the smartest thing to do, you will see.

(*Continued*)

Composite Vignette 8.3. (*Continued*)

It will solve all the problems. We are using the smarts of private sector catastrophic insurance."

The head of a bilateral foreign aid agency worried that the Kawanda Network for Disease Control and Prevention could prevent his country's Centers for Disease Control and Prevention from continuing to ship biological samples from Kawanda without the consent of governments across Kawanda, and without Kawandan scientists having the first say in how biological samples from their own countries would be taken, handled, analyzed, and reported upon. Several of his peers agreed. "They don't need a Kawanda Network. We should continue doing it for them!"

For the first time that anyone could remember, Coumba lost her preternatural calm. She tore into Stevens and his acolytes. "How dare you, an entitled and smug bunch of North Americans and Europeans, arrogate to yourselves the divine right to dictate what Kawandans can and should do, and what we cannot and should not do? Let me be clear: there will be a viable Kawanda Network for Disease Control and Prevention, with or without your support. And if I ever hear any of you claim that you were always for it, I will set you straight in the most public way possible. Shame on you, all of you. Now, if you will excuse me, I must leave for the airport."

The meeting ended in confusion.

Stevens had a follow-up meeting with Edgar Rogerson, CEO of the Alliance for Global Health. It was their first one-on-one breakfast meeting since the Meloba outbreak in West Kawanda in 2014–2016. Rogerson had not forgiven Stevens's conduct, which he, Rogerson, considered to be one of showboating and gratuitously scoring points at the expense of the Alliance for Global Health. Stevens stood his ground. "You people made a mess of it. But you know how much I respect you. Let's agree to disagree and move forward." That was when Rick McAllister of the New York Tribune walked to their table. With a wry smile, he said "Good morning. Multiple sources tell me there is a big kerfuffle over whether to finance and support the Kawanda Network for Disease Control and Prevention. My sources say that you, Mr. Stevens, have refused to put any funds into it and that you, Mr. Rogerson, want to control and suffocate it because you see it as a threat to your mandate. What is going on?" Stevens and Rogerson declined to comment.

(Continued)

Composite Vignette 8.3. (*Continued*)

Two days later, the New York Tribune published a front-page story by McAllister. It was a detailed account of the lack of leadership, institutional ossification, unresponsiveness, turfism, and inter-agency bickering, with sources speaking on condition of anonymity for fear of retribution. In a highly unusual move, the Tribune followed up with a sobering editorial, published on November 26, 2019:

"The World Development Fund, by its own Articles of Agreement, must invest in projects that yield the highest return on investment compared to others. How many other projects can claim to potentially avert a multi-trillion dollar economic collapse that would arise from a terrible pandemic? That is the projected benefit of the Kawanda Network for Disease Control and Prevention. Yet, Mr. Jack Stevens, CEO of the World Development Fund, is hostile to precisely that investment.

Anyone who spends any time with Stevens knows that he cannot finish any meeting without waxing poetic that the arc of the moral universe is long and bends toward justice. But he is not living up to that creed. It is an open secret that instead of doing the right thing by investing in the Kawanda Network for Disease Control and Prevention, Stevens is touting a vanity project called the Pandemic Urgency Fund (PUF). Serious economists outside the World Development Fund have concluded that the PUF is a comical construct. But Stevens, his Chief Director for Health, and his Principal Economist for Kawanda persist in this folly. In fact, they have doubled down on the PUF.

Let us be clear. The main reason for foot dragging by the World Development Fund and its sycophantic cabal is that the idea originated from the Heads of State of Kawanda. Had it been proposed by some minions in one of the G7 countries, Stevens and his ilk would be running around to make it happen as part of the hollow rituals of global initiatives to Save Kawanda.

It does not take much to imagine a devastating pandemic overwhelming the continent of Kawanda. Imagine the crippling effect on the global economy, imperiling lives, and livelihoods. If that happens, blame not the Heads of State of Kawanda, who have

(*Continued*)

Composite Vignette 8.3. (*Continued*)

taken the initiative. Blame the World Development Fund, which prefers the vanity project called PUF to a badly needed one, and the Alliance for Global Health, whose claims to mandates far exceed its capacity to do anything useful."

Two weeks later, in December 2019, Stevens and McAllister reluctantly announced a formal agreement that included financing and technical cooperation for the Kawanda Network for Disease Control and Prevention. One month later, a panicky Alliance for Global Health declared that an outbreak of a newly discovered hemorrhagic virus, GUNSET-20, had become both a pandemic and a Public Health Emergency of International Concern.

Much of DAH is due for a thorough overhaul. There is a pressing need to do better, and a break from ossified narratives and practices of DAH is central to such improvements. Potential directions for changes and improvements are considered in the concluding chapter.

References

[1] Xu K, Soucat A, Kutzin J *et al.* 2019. Global spending on health: A world in transition. *World Health Organization.* pp. 11–13. https://www.who.int/health_financing/documents/health-expenditure-report-2019/en/. Accessed on March 17, 2021.

[2] Dieleman J, Micah A, Murray C. 2019. Global health spending and development assistance for health. *JAMA*, 321(21): 2073–2074. Accessed on March 17, 2021.

[3] Global Burden of Disease Health Financing Collaborating Network. 2019. Past, present, and future of global health financing: a review of development assistance, government, out-of-pocket, and other private spending on health for 195 countries, 1995–2050. *The Lancet*, 393(10187): 2233–2260. Accessed on March 17, 2021.

[4] Global Burden of Disease Health Financing Collaborating Network. 2020. Health sector spending and spending on HIV/AIDS, tuberculosis, and malaria, and development assistance for health: progress towards Sustainable Development Goal 3. *The Lancet*, 396(10252): 693–724. https://doi.org/10.1016/S0140-6736(20)30608-5. Accessed on March 17, 2021.

[5] Deileman JL, Schenider MT, Haakenstad A *et al.* 2016. Development assistance for health: past trends, associations, and the future of international financial flows for health. *The Lancet*, 387(10037): 2536–2544. https://www.thelancet.com/journals/lancet/article/PIIS0140-6736(16)30168-4/fulltext. Accessed on March 17, 2021.

[6] Micah A, Zlavog B, Friedman S, Reynolds A *et al.* 2017. The US provided $13 billion in development assistance for health in 2016, less per person than many peer nations. *Health Affairs*, 36(12). https://www.healthaffairs.org/doi/full/10.1377/hlthaff.2017.1055. Accessed on March 11, 2021.

[7] McKee C, Blampied C, Mitchell I, Rogerson A. 2020. Revisiting aid effectiveness: a new framework and set of measures for assessing aid "quality." Center for Global Development. https://www.cgdev.org/publication/revisiting-aid-effectiveness-new-framework-and-set-measures-assessing-aid. Accessed on March 11, 2021.

[8] The Independent Panel for Pandemic Preparedness and Response. COVID-19: Make it the last pandemic. https://theindependentpanel.org/wp-content/uploads/2021/05/COVID-19-Make-it-the-Last-Pandemic_final.pdf. Accessed on May 13, 2021.

[9] World Bank. 2019. Pandemic emergency financing facility. https://www.worldbank.org/en/topic/pandemics/brief/pandemic-emergency-financing-facility. Accessed on May 17, 2021.

[10] Schäferhoff M, Fewer S, Kraus J, Richter E, Summers LH *et al.* 2015. How much donor financing for health is channelled to global versus country-specific aid functions? *The Lancet*, 386: 2436–2441. https://www.thelancet.com/journals/lancet/article/PIIS0140-6736(15)61161-8/fulltext. Accessed on June 9, 2021.

[11] Schäferhoff M, Chodavadia P, Martinez S, McDade KK, Fewer S *et al.* 2019. International funding for global common goods for health: An analysis using the creditor reporting system and G-FINDER databases. *Health Systems & Reform,* 5(4): 350–365. https://www.tandfonline.com/doi/full/10.1080/23288604.2019.16 63646. Accessed on June 9, 2021.

[12] Martinez Alvarez M, Acharya A, Arregoces L, Bearley L. Trends in the alignment and harmonization of reproductive, maternal, newborn, and child health funding, 2008–13. *Health Affairs*, 36(11). https://www.healthaffairs.org/doi/10.1377/hlthaff.2017.0364. Accessed on March 11, 2021.

[13] High Level Forum. 2005. Paris declaration on aid effectiveness http://www.oecd.org/dac/effectiveness/parisdeclarationandaccraagendaforaction.htm. Accessed on March 11, 2021.

[14] Mitchell I, Calleja R, Hughes S. 2021. The quality of official development assistance. Center for Global Development. https://www.cgdev.org/publication/quality-official-development-assistance. Accessed on May 25, 2021.

[15] Packard RM. 2016. *A History of Global Health. Interventions into the Lives of Other Peoples.* Baltimore, MD: Johns Hopkins University Press. pp. 13–46.

[16] World Health Organization. How WHO is funded. https://www.who.int/about/funding. Accessed on May 28, 2021.

[17] Aso T. 2017. Crucial role of finance ministry in achieving universal health coverage. *The Lancet,* 390(10111): 2415–2417. https://www.thelancet.com/journals/lancet/article/PIIS0140-6736(17)33077-5/fulltext. Accessed on March 11, 2021.

[18] Shiozaki Y, Philpott J, Touraine M, Grohe G, Lorenzin B, Hunt J *et al.* G7 health ministers' Kobe Communiqué. https://www.thelancet.com/journals/lancet/article/PIIS0140-6736(16)31663-4/fulltext. Accessed on March 11, 2021.

[19] Bureau of the Chairperson. 2020. Statement on AU vaccines financing strategy. https://au.int/ar/node/39545. Accessed on March 11, 2021.

[20] Fenner F, Henderson DA, Arita I *et al.* 1988. *Smallpox and its Eradication.* World Health Organization. https://apps.who.int/iris/handle/10665/39485. Accessed on March 12, 2021.

[21] World Health Organization. African Programme for Onchocerciasis Control (APOC). https://www.who.int/blindness/partnerships/APOC/en/ Accessed on March 11, 2021.

[22] Lucas AO. 2010. *It Was the Best of Times. From Local to Global Health.* Ibadan, Nigeria: Book Builders. pp. 216–225.

[23] World Health Organization. About the WHO framework convention on tobacco control. https://www.who.int/fctc/about/en/. Accessed on March 18, 2021.

[24] Atun R, de Jongh T, Secci F, Ohiri K, Adeyi O. 2010. A systematic review of the evidence on integration of targeted health interventions into health systems. *Health Policy and Planning,* 25(1): 1–14. https://doi.org/10.1093/heapol/czp053. Accessed on June 9, 2021

[25] Atun R, de Jongh T, Secci F, Ohiri K, Adeyi O. 2010. Integration of targeted health interventions into health systems: a conceptual framework for analysis. *Health Policy and Planning,* 25(2): 104–111, https://doi.org/10.1093/heapol/czp055. Accessed on March 18, 2021.

[26] Newell KH. 1988. Selective primary health care: The counter revolution. *Social Science & Medicine,* 26(9): 903–906. https://www.sciencedirect.com/science/article/abs/pii/0277953688904091. Accessed on March 20, 2021.

[27] Biesma R, Brugha R, Harmer A *et al.* 2009. The effects of global health initiatives on country health systems: A review of the evidence from HIV/AIDS control. *Health Policy Plan.* 24(4): 239–252. doi: 10.1093/heapol/czp025. Accessed on March 21, 2021.

[28] Mwisongo A, Nabyonga-Orem J. 2016. Global health initiatives in Africa — governance, priorities, harmonisation and alignment. *BMC Health Services Research.* 16(Suppl 4): 212. doi: 10.1186/s12913-016-1448-9. Accessed on March 11, 2021.

[29] Piva P, Dodd R. 2009. Where did all the aid go? An in-depth analysis of increased health aid flows over the past 10 years. *Bulletin of the World Health Organization*, 87: 930–939. doi: 10.2471/BLT.08.058677. Accessed on March 11, 2021.

[30] Vaillancourt D. 2009. Do health sector-wide approaches achieve results? : Emerging evidence and lessons from six countries. IEG Working Paper; 2009/4. Washington, DC: World Bank. http://hdl.handle.net/10986/28064. Accessed on March 11, 2021.

[31] World Health Organization. 2007. *Everybody Business: Strengthening Health Systems to Improve Health Outcomes: WHO's Framework for Action.* Geneva. https://www.who.int/healthsystems/strategy/en/. Accessed on March 17, 2021.

[32] IEG Review Team. 2018. *Bangladesh — BD: Health Sector Development Program (English).* Washington, D.C.: World Bank Group. https://documents. worldbank.org/en/publication/documents-reports/documentdetail/ 114181528922648368/bangladesh-bd-health-sector-development-program. Accessed on March 11, 2021.

[33] Ahsan KZ, Streatfield PK, Ijdi R, Escudero GM *et al.* 2016. Fifteen years of sector-wide approach (SWAp) in Bangladesh health sector: an assessment of progress. *Health Policy and Planning*, 31(5), 612–623, https://doi.org/10.1093/ heapol/czv108. Accessed on March 11, 2021.

[34] World Health Organization. A guide to WHO's role in sector-wide approaches to health development. https://www.who.int/hdp/publications/swaps_guide.pdf. Accessed on March 18, 2021.

[35] Peters D, Paina L, Schleimann F. 2013. Sector-wide approaches (SWAps) in health: what have we learned? *Health Policy and Planning*, 28(8): 884–890, https://doi.org/10.1093/heapol/czs128. Accessed on March 18, 2021.

[36] World Bank. 2002. Implementation completion report (TF-20967; IDA-26600) on a credit in the amount of SDR 38.7 million (USD 56 million equivalent) to the Republic of Zambia for the Health Sector Support Project. http://documents1.

worldbank.org/curated/en/433381468781197885/pdf/multi0page.pdf. Accessed on March 18, 2021.

[37] World Bank. Ghana Health Sector Support Project. Implementation completion report review. Operations Evaluation Department. Report Number: ICRR11541.2003. http://documents1.worldbank.org/curated/en/126151475082409088/pdf/ 000020051-20140612070900.pdf. Accessed on March 18, 2021.

[38] World Bank. Second Health Sector Program Support Project. Implementation completion review report. Independent Evaluation Group. Report Number: ICRR12848. http://documents1.worldbank.org/curated/en/536391474590718007/ pdf/000020051-20140618084609.pdf. Accessed on March 18, 2021.

[39] The Lancet Global Health. Global health 2021: Who tells the story? 9(2). https://www.thelancet.com/journals/langlo/article/piis2214-109x(21)00004-8/ fulltext. Accessed on March 11, 2021.

[40] Abimbola S, Pai M. 2020. Will global health survive its decolonization? *The Lancet.* 396(10263): 1627–1828. https://www.thelancet.com/journals/lancet/ article/PIIS0140-6736(20)32417-X/fulltext. Accessed on March 11, 2021.

[41] Yerramilli P. To decolonize global health, we must examine the global political economy. Think Global Health. https://www.thinkglobalhealth.org/article/ decolonize-global-health-we-must-examine-global-political-economy. Accessed on March 11, 2021.

[42] Velin L, Lartigue J, Johnson S *et al.* Conference equity in global health: A systematic review of factors impacting LMIC representation at global health conferences. *BMJ Global Health.* https://gh.bmj.com/content/6/1/e003455. Accessed on March 11, 2021.

[43] Shiffman J. Knowledge, moral claims and the exercise of power in global health. 10.15171/ijhpm.2014.120. Accessed on March 11, 2021.

[44] Pai M. 2020. Global health technologies: Time to re-think the 'trickle down' model. https://www.forbes.com/sites/madhukarpai/2020/02/17/global-health-technologies-time-to-re-think-the-trickle-down-model/?sh=1e8e1ed144d9. Accessed on March 11, 2021.

[45] Jumbam D. 2020. How not to write about global health. *BMJ.* https://gh.bmj. com/content/5/7/e003164. Accessed on March 11, 2021.

[46] Nordling L. 2021. US malaria project attacked as scientific colonialism. https://www.researchprofessionalnews.com/rr-news-africa-pan-african-2021-2-us-malaria-project-attacked-as-scientific-colonialism/. Accessed on March 11, 2021.

[47] Abimbola S, Asthana S, Cortes CM, Guinto RR, Jumbam DT *et al.* 2021. Addressing power asymmetries in global health: Imperatives in the wake of the

COVID-19 pandemic. *PLoS Medicine.* https://doi.org/10.1371/journal. pmed.1003604. Accessed on April 30, 2021.

[48] Hochschild A. 1999. *King Leopold's Ghost. A Story of Greed, Terror, and Heroism in Colonial Africa.* First Mariner Books.

[49] Burke, J. 2020. Belgium must return tooth of murdered Congolese leader, judge rules. *The Guardian.* https://www.theguardian.com/world/2020/sep/10/judge-orders-return-of-tooth-said-to-be-from-assassinated-congolese-icon. Accessed on May 26, 2021.

[50] Palca J, Lichtman F. 2011. *Annoying. The Science of What Bugs Us.* New Jersey: John Wiley & Sons, Inc.

[51] Ritchie H. 2021.Western countries prevented African nations from having their own vaccine. Vice. https://www.vice.com/en/article/epnxd7/africa-covid-vaccine-blocked-by-western-countries. Accessed on May 14, 2021.

[52] Okonjo-Iweala N. 2012. *Reforming the Unreformable: Lessons from Nigeria.* Cambridge, MA: MIT Press. p. 131.

[53] Atun R, Aydın S, Chakraborty S *et al.* 2013. Universal health coverage in Turkey: enhancement of equity. *The Lancet,* 382: 65–99. http://dx.doi.org/10.1016/S0140-6736(13)61051-X. Accessed on March 15, 2021.

[54] El-Akel W, El-Sayed M, Kassas M. 2017. National treatment program of hepatitis C in Egypt: Hepatitis C virus model of care. *Journal of Viral Hepatitis.* https://doi.org/10.1111/jvh.12668. Accessed on March 15, 2021.

[55] Workie N, Ramana GNV. 2013. The health extension program in Ethiopia. UNICO Studies Series; No. 10. World Bank, Washington, DC. https://openknowledge.worldbank.org/handle/10986/13280. Accessed on March 15, 2021.

[56] Gosis J, Arbeloa P, Romo Sanchez A *et al.* 2020. *Study of Hospital Concessions in Chile: Reimbursable Advisory Services* (Vol. 2). https://documents.worldbank.org/en/publication/documents-reports/documentdetail/713621603953300310/executive-summary. Accessed on March 15, 2021.

[57] World Bank. 2018. Healthy China: Deepening health reform by building high-quality and value-based service delivery. https://www.worldbank.org/en/results/2018/04/16/healthy-china-deepening-health-reform-by-building-high-quality-value-based-service-delivery. Accessed on March 15, 2021.

[58] Denny C. 2002. The contended malcontent. https://www.theguardian.com/business/2002/jul/06/globalisation. Accessed on March 9, 2021.

Chapter 9

GPS for Wise Investments in Global Health

"The maker of an implement, therefore, has a correct belief about its merits and defects, but he is obliged to get this by associating with and listening to someone who knows. And the person with the relevant knowledge is the user."

—Plato, *The Republic*[a]

"Very well, since you insist, I will give you my opinion."

—Ismail Kadare[b]

Synopsis

This concluding chapter is a synopsis of key messages for investors who seek to maximize returns in terms of health and institutional impacts. The preceding chapters explored the conceptual and operational premise of global health, real-world examples of global health in practice, and multiple dimensions of its interface with DAH. While readers will have different perspectives on any single aspect of the book, I hope that all will agree on one thing: global health is very complex in real life.

---

[a]Plato. 1955. *The Republic*. Translated with an introduction by Desmond Lee. Penguin Books. p. 368.
[b]Kadare I. 1986. *The General of the Dead Army*. Quartet Books. p. 145.

But complexity is not an excuse for paralysis amidst vast unmet needs for health services, inequities in the capacities and capabilities of health systems, and dysfunctional approaches to DAH. In the quest for better performance, investors optimizing for enduring health and institutional impacts, equity, solidarity between the Global North and the Global South, and self-reliance by the Global South have multiple levers that are mutually reinforcing.

9.1. Clarity of Purpose

The complex and often conflicting agendas at the roots of colonial, international, and global health can trip up even those enterprises with the best of intentions. Additionally, because the needs are so vast and the means so complex, it is easy to be very busy but without clarity of purpose in contemporary global health. Therefore, policy makers, influencers, and practitioners should make a serious effort to ensure clarity of purpose. What are they seeking to achieve, where, how, why, and on whose terms? These seem like very basic questions, but all too often they are not addressed, which lays the foundation for catastrophic failures.

9.2. Primacy of Recipient Country and Regional Interests

The asymmetry of financial and institutional power between the Global North and the Global South all too often causes global health enterprises to proceed with a default setting in which the Global North makes the rules, plays the game, and referees the game. This is inherently bad, regardless of any party's good intentions. Progress requires both self-awareness and humility on the part of the Global North, and more self-funded assertiveness by the Global South, to flip the script: the explicit basis for engagement should be the interests of countries whose policies and programs are under discussion. The need is high for explicit agreements on policy and program objectives and counterfactuals.

A recap of key points from the chapter on the strategic and geopolitical lessons from COVID-19 is in order here. It is important to overhaul the International Health Regulations (IHR), with greater attention to strategic incentives and less reliance on lofty but unenforceable norms and regulations. Investments in Country and Regional Institutions and Networks will benefit both the host countries — or regions — and others. Finally, governments should reconsider the old orthodoxies and make strategic investments in the industrial production of goods needed for preventing and responding to large disease outbreaks.

9.3. Emphasis on Learning

Hubris and aversion to learning undermine the relevance of policies and the effectiveness of programs. It is prudent for all parties to place expected learning close to the top of the agenda. Such learning includes knowing what, knowing how, and knowing why some things work and others don't. It is not as easy as it might sound; such learning is bound to disrupt the comfort zones of established practitioners within countries and the default power equilibrium between foreign agencies and country leaders.

9.4. Overhauling Legacy Foreign Aid Paradigms

Both bilateral and multilateral types of foreign aid need a rethink. The multilateral construct has some checks and balances from multiple perspectives but is still prone to the comfort of groupthink. The bilateral construct is especially fraught with unchecked risks of rich countries dictating to poorer countries and bullying those multilateral institutions that depend on their financial clout. Both need to change.

The spectrum of DAH currently does far too many things across LICs and LMICs. There are some successes, and credit for these go — in various combinations and with varying degrees of clarity — to the beneficiary countries, their governments, financiers of DAH, and intermediary agencies, both domestic and foreign. Such successes merit continuation and modification in line with country realities and fiscal constraints. At the same time, the global health and DAH landscapes are full of modalities, interventions, and business models of dubious usefulness, and a reckoning is long overdue.[1] More tinkering will not do, and neither will an escalation of commitment to failing or mediocre approaches. A few fundamental changes to DAH for global health would better serve beneficiary countries while providing ample transparency for financiers and beneficiaries alike.

9.5. End Foreign Aid for Basic Health Inputs in LICs and LMICs

The first shift is for external financiers to end all foreign aid or development assistance for the most essential inputs for basic health services — such as vaccines for routine childhood immunizations, insecticide-treated bednets for the prevention of malaria, items on WHO's Model List of Essential Medicines, and other basic medical supplies and supply chain management. These items are so highly cost effective and the need for them is so predictable that they should be elementary responsibilities for the countries themselves. This proposition converges with a key argument of the Lancet Commission on Investing in Health, which was chaired by former United States Treasury Secretary Lawrence Summers.[2]

An abrupt cessation is neither sensible nor appropriate in practice. One option for a target date is the year 2030, based on the premise that on September 25, 2015, "the resolution on Transforming our world: the 2030 Agenda for Sustainable Development (A/RES/70/1) adopted the target of universal health coverage by 2030, including financial risk protection, access to quality essential health-care services and access to safe, effective, quality and affordable essential medicines and vaccines for all."[3] LICs and LMICs would have several years to prepare for this scenario, which would concentrate the minds of policy makers and influencers on the need to truly and finally take responsibility for the most basic health services in their own countries. This transition might involve up to 76% of current DAH, based on recent estimates for country-specific functions.[4]

International financiers who insist on financing such inputs have a path: they should subsidize such commodities at the global or regional level and leave it to the countries to manage the procurement of commodities, either by themselves or through their procurement agents. Even if country budgets remained constant from one year to the next, the purchasing power would increase because of the supranational subsidy for such commodities. This approach would also benefit the only reasonable exceptions — countries in situations of active conflict with displaced or underserved populations.

Financing the most basic inputs from domestic sources is a demonstration of governments taking responsibility for the needs of their own populations.

External financiers should leave it to countries to organize the procurement of those inputs via the public and private sectors. Such procurement would be in the full glare of public scrutiny.

9.6. Refocus Foreign Aid on the Most Complex Strategic Reforms and Institutional Development

There is no extraordinary complexity in procuring and delivering products like insecticide-treated bednets. The problem is that a self-perpetuating Development Industrial Complex has developed around them, with a strong incentive for countries to continue patterns of dependency on DAH, and purveyors of DAH are comfortable with recycling the same programs with different labels. Where foreign aid could add value is in the conceptualization, design, and implementation support for solutions to complex challenges of structural reforms of hospital systems, laboratory networks, research networks, insurance systems, country-level institutions for strategic management, intelligent purchasing of services, health technology assessment and application, and public goods (by improving country and regional institutions for disease surveillance and response capacities to prevent and respond to epidemics and pandemics).

A shift in focus also means rethinking the premise of approaches such as Performance-Based Financing[5,6] and Cash-On Delivery.[7] Performance and incentives would shift from menial and micro concerns of end-line service delivery to mission-critical functions of Southern systems, Southern institutions, and their employees, for without those institutions, investments by Northern financiers are unlikely to have durable impact.

9.7. Reform Technical Assistance to Ensure Fitness for Purpose

The traditional approaches to donor-funded technical assistance fall into three broad categories.

(1) Type 1: For those financed by bilateral financiers of the Global North, the selection of technical service providers is mostly determined by the financiers. Recipient countries have generally modest say, if any, in the criteria and selection process.

(2) Type 2: For those financed from the proceeds of grants, credits, or loans from development banks, the borrower countries generally conduct the selection according to publicly available guidelines for the procurement of services from individuals and firms.

(3) Type 3: Technical assistance provided by large NGOs of Northern origin tends to be tightly controlled by those NGOs and is thus much closer to Type 1 than Type 2.

Types 1 and 3 have the serious deficiency of asymmetry of information between financiers and beneficiaries. There is a risk that financiers, even if unwittingly, foist upon recipient countries some providers of technical assistance that are not only irrelevant to local needs and realities but could leave the recipients worse off than they might have been without the technical assistance.

The USAID's and US-PMI's approach to development financing is the epitome of bad practice in its egregious aversion to real capacity building — and in its willful resistance to leadership by country institutions in the Global South, which are relegated to playing gofer roles for American contractors. For example, in January 2021, US-PMI launched a five-year, US\$30 million operational research and program evaluation project. The project would be led by a United States-based contractor in collaboration with seven other organizations based in the United States, the United Kingdom, and Australia. After decades of purportedly building capacity in malaria-endemic countries, USAID and US-PMI could not find any African institution worthy of taking the lead in that operational and program evaluation project. The project has been roundly — and fittingly — condemned as "scientific colonialism"[8] and for perpetuating "structural inequities."[9] Highly qualified professionals in the Global South, many of whom know the subject matter and operational realities better than their counterparts from the Global North, are repeatedly confined to playing roles reminiscent of *Hidden Figures*,[10] only for others to take the glory. In the 2021 edition of the Quality of Official Development

Assistance (QuODA),[11] the United States unsurprisingly was in the bottom half of providers for Prioritization, Ownership, and Evaluation. The ill-conceived business model of USAID and US-PMI, which is funded by taxpayers, continues without reform. A change is long overdue.[12] According to the Office of Inspector General at USAID:[13]

> *"USAID implements nearly all of its activities through contracts (acquisition) or grants (assistance). OIG's audit on USAID's award management found that insufficient oversight of awards has resulted in USAID not fully assessing implementers' performance and holding them accountable for achieving results, calling into question whether the Agency adequately protects taxpayer funds."*

Type 1 approach to foreign aid also features some astonishing acts of incompetence that are hard to justify, and which render any defense of the *status quo* as nothing more than a homage to the rent-seeking Development Industrial Complex.[14]

Many external counterparts from the Global North, who provide "technical assistance" to parties in the Global South, truly bring expertise to their work. However, many others from the Global North are either mediocre or plainly incompetent. Many are ill-suited for responsibilities that require a combination of deep knowledge of the subject, breadth of know-how, and policy wisdom. Especially when such technical assistance comes from bilaterally funded programs, country officials are typically not empowered to decline them, for fear of annoying donors and losing funds that are tied to the technical assistance.

One solution is for all foreign aid financing technical assistance to be in the form of a draw-down fund and linked to an open-access roster of technical experts. Recipient government officials and institutions, not the Global North financiers of technical assistance, would prepare the selection criteria and conduct the competitive selection process to procure technical services from individuals and institutions. Depending on the size of the contract, the bilateral agencies funding the work program would have the right to object to the selection and would specify in the public domain their reasons for objecting to any selection process or its outcome. The results would be in the public domain as contributions to transparency and accountability.

9.8. Support Mission-Critical Institutions at Country and Regional Levels

Much of the reason for the continued use of foreign technical experts derives from weaknesses in country and regional institutions of LICs and MICs. The medium-term solution is for donors from the Global North to put themselves out of business in a constructive way, by vigorously supporting the development of Global South institutions that can perform effectively.

This would take some shifts in thinking. For example, instead of investing in more Northern centers of excellence to provide services to the Global South,[15] donors should invest in Southern institutions and centers of excellence across a range of functions: basic research in the health sciences; policy analysis via Southern think tanks; support for government departments of planning, research, and statistics; heavy investments in institutions for disease surveillance and response to disease outbreaks; and in schools of public health, operations management, and health economics. This requires serious commitment to gritty partnerships and deliberately structured financing, of which there are some examples.[16]

Models of development assistance that see countries as the sole unit of analysis and engagement risk fast becoming irrelevant, especially in regional and global public goods. Accordingly, it is important to expand and customize development assistance that supports regional and subregional centers for disease prevention, surveillance, and control. COVID-19 has laid bare the risks to the Global South of continued reliance on the Global North for supplies of crucial products like diagnostics, medicines, and vaccines. These are areas that merit local production in the Global South, whose governments and regional institutions should prioritize public–private partnerships to meet their own needs.

Two examples of relevant institutions merit attention here. One is the Africa CDC, the plucky new institution that featured in Chapter 2 of this book. An older example is The Special Program for Research and Training in Tropical Diseases (TDR), "a global program of scientific collaboration that helps facilitate, support and influence efforts to combat diseases of poverty." Cosponsored by UNICEF, UNDP, the World Bank, and WHO,[17] TDR has made enormous contributions to product development for the control of several otherwise neglected diseases that afflict the poor in the Global South, and it has developed scientific research capacity across the world. Establishing and running collaborative institutions and programs at the global or regional level can be very challenging. Despite the challenges, such institutions and collaborations, if set up with a clear sense of purpose and if well led, yield high returns on investment.

9.9. Requiem for Neo-dependency

Investors need to recognize that while the legacy of colonization persists, an even greater problem is that of neo-dependency. The changes outlined in this chapter would compel actors across the spectrum of global health to focus more clearly on their comparative advantages and to justify their continued existence based on what they can contribute, not on the basis of historical mandates or just because they come to the table with a lot of money. Crucially, these changes would compel policy makers and governments of LICs and MICs to exercise their agency and take responsibility for what they should.

Development assistance is prone to gaming by financiers — for purposes including but not limited to institutional self-perpetuation, politically smooth relations with beneficiary countries, and staff under pressure to meet targets for grants, credits, or loans. It is also prone to gaming by recipients — for purposes that include increasing short-term revenues regardless of long-term consequences, politically smooth relations with donors, and aversion to precisely the challenging decisions needed for long-term success. This gaming needs to be called out wherever it exists. Foreign donors should aim to put themselves out of the business of endlessly paying, or pretending to pay, for the most basic inputs for primary health care, and graduate into value-adding support for very complex institutional development, systemic reforms, and public goods at the regional and global levels. It is past time for the Global South to leave behind its self-entrapment in neo-dependency. A brighter future is possible.

References

[1] *The New York Times*. Foreign aid is having a reckoning. https://www.nytimes.com/2021/02/13/opinion/africa-foreign-aid-philanthropy.html. Accessed on March 20, 2021.

[2] Jamison DT, Summers LH, Alleyne G, Arrow KJ, Berkley S *et al*. 2013. Global health 2035: A world converging within a generation. *The Lancet*, 9908: 1898–1955. https://www.thelancet.com/journals/lancet/issue/vol382no9908/PIIS0140-6736(13)X6061-1. Accessed on June 9, 2021.

[3] United Nations. International universal health coverage day, 12 December. https://www.un.org/en/observances/universal-health-coverage-day/background#:~:text=On%2025%20September%202015%2C%20the,safe%2C%20effective%2C%20quality%20and%20affordable. Accessed on February 22, 2021.

[4] Schäferhoff M, Chodavadia P, Martinez S, McDade KK, Fewer S *et al*. 2019. International funding for global common goods for health: an analysis using the creditor reporting system and G-FINDER databases. 2019. *Health Systems & Reform*, 5(4): 350–365. https://www.tandfonline.com/doi/full/10.1080/23288604.2019.1663646. Accessed on June 9, 2021.

[5] World Health Organization. Performance-based financing. https://www.who.int/health_financing/topics/performance-based-financing/en/. Accessed on March 20, 2021.

[6] Paul E, Renmans D. 2018. Performance-based financing in the heath sector in low- and middle-income countries: Is there anything whereof it may be said, see, this is new? *International Journal of Health Planning and Management*, 33(1): 51–66. https://onlinelibrary.wiley.com/doi/abs/10.1002/hpm.2409. Accessed on March 20, 2021.

[7] Center for Global Development. Cash On Delivery. https://www.cgdev.org/topics/cash-on-delivery. Accessed on March 20, 2021.

[8] Nordling L. 2021. US malaria project attacked as 'scientific colonialism.' https://www.researchprofessionalnews.com/rr-news-africa-pan-african-2021-2-us-malaria-project-attacked-as-scientific-colonialism/. Accessed on April 15, 2021.

[9] Erondu N, Aniebo I, Kyobutungi C, Midega J, Okiro E, Okomu F. 2021. Open letter to international funders of science and development in Africa. *Nature Medicine*. https://www.nature.com/articles/s41591-021-01307-8. Accessed on April 15, 2021.

[10] Shetterly ML. 2016. Hidden Figures: The American Dream and the Untold Story of the Black Women Mathematicians Who Helped Win the Space Race. London: William Collins.

[11] Mitchell I, Calleja R, Hughes S. 2021. The quality of official development assistance. *Center for Global Development.* https://www.cgdev.org/publication/quality-official-development-assistance. Accessed on May 25, 2021.

[12] Kerr W, Guzdar M. 2021. USAID's Big Contracts Don't Pay Off. *Foreign Policy.* https://foreignpolicy.com/2021/05/18/usaid-biden-power-contracts-money-procurement/. Accessed on July 29, 2021.

[13] USAID Office of Inspector General. 2021. Office of Inspector General Semiannual Report to Congress April 1, 2019-September 30, 2019. Washington DC. USAID. Page 10. https://oig.usaid.gov/sites/default/files/2019-11/USAID%20OIG%20Semi%20Annual%20Report%20to%20Congress%20-%20October%2030%2C%202019.pdf. Accessed on July 29, 2021.

[14] Welsh T. 2018. 'Significant mistakes' in USAID global health supply chain, House says. Devex. https://www.devex.com/news/significant-mistakes-in-usaid-global-health-supply-chain-house-says-93674. Accessed on March 20, 2021.

[15] Schwab T. Are Bill Gates's billions distorting public health data? *The Nation.* https://www.thenation.com/article/society/gates-covid-data-ihme/. Accessed on March 20, 2021.

[16] World Bank. Building centers of excellence in Africa to address regional development challenges. https://www.worldbank.org/en/results/2020/10/14/building-centers-of-excellence-in-africa-to-address-regional-development-challenges. Accessed on March 20, 2021.

[17] TDR. https://tdr.who.int/about-us. Accessed on June 9, 2021.

Index

World Scientific Series in Health Investment and Financing

(Continued from page ii)

Forthcoming

Financing Universal Access to Healthcare: A Comparative Review of Incremental Health Insurance Reforms in the OECD
Alexander S. Preker

Capital Finance in the Health Industry: A User Manual for Investors and Companies
Alexander S. Preker and Les Funtleyder

Handbook on Health System Financing and Organization
Dov Chernichovsky

How Health Aid Meets the Challenge of Mixed Health Systems: Reluctant Partners
April Harding

Printed in the United States
by Baker & Taylor Publisher Services